Run Simple

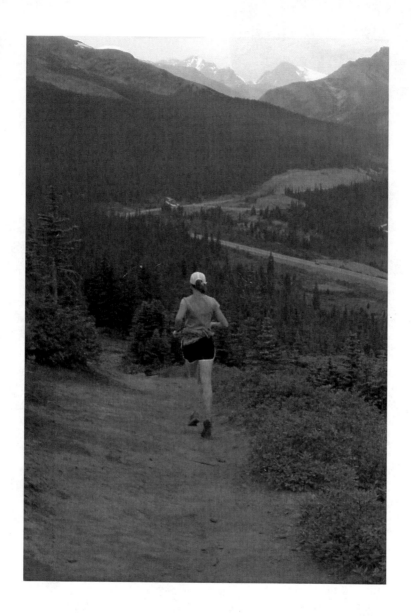

Run
Simple

A Minimalist Approach
to Fitness and Well-Being

Duncan Larkin

WESTHOLME
Yardley

Westholme Publishing, LLC
904 Edgewood Road
Yardley, Pennsylvania 19067
Visit our Web site at www.westholmepublishing.com

First Printing June 2012
10 9 8 7 6 5 4 3 2 1

ISBN: 978-1-59416-162-9

Also available as an eBook.

Printed in the United States of America.

Contents

Acknowledgments

This page is usually the place in a book where the author thanks certain people in his life—people who were instrumental in making the book possible. I would like to continue with this convention, but instead of just listing a series of names, I'd like to instead offer a bit more detail so that everyone but the person being thanked doesn't skip this part of the book.

To Erin Jackson: It's hard enough living with an obsessive runner; it's even harder living with one who writes books. Thank you for putting up with me.

To my parents, Don and Marilyn Larkin: Thank you for continuing to teach me how to love unconditionally.

To my agent, Rich Henshaw: Over the years, I've received hundreds of literary agency rejection letters, but one of them didn't come from you. Thank you for believing in me and in *Run Simple*.

To Bruce H. Franklin at Westholme: Thank you for your interest in this important concept and for ultimately deciding to publish this book.

To Mario Fraioli: Thank you for giving the manuscript a good run-through.

To Toby Tanser, Lauren Fleshman, Brad Hudson, and Anton Krupicka: Thank you for donating your valuable time and ideas to this book.

To Amy Schramm: Thank you for demonstrating the sample exercises.

And finally, to you, the loyal runner, that thoroughly dedicated person who heads out the door in the middle of a rainstorm to pound pavement: Thank you for picking up this book. I hope it gets you to change at least one thing about your running. If it does, I've succeeded and so will you.

Simply Running

ARE YOU A SATISFIED RUNNER? If you're reading this book, then there's a good chance you aren't, or you want more out of running. There's a reason you have picked it up and begun thumbing through it; you've made that valuable investment of your time and hard-earned money into running and you want to get something out of it.

You want to run faster; you want to feel better.

This probably isn't your first running book. I'll wager you've read plenty of how-to articles in various running magazines as well. And there's no doubt whatsoever that you're no stranger to searching for running tips on the Web. I'm quite sure you've been to a running bulletin board or two and that you've wandered around many a prerace expo in search of something (anything!) that will help you break that stubborn, 10-year-old 5K personal record.

You want to improve.

After all, what's the point of repetitive, day-in and day-out running if not to get better at it—to find out how good you really can get at this sport?

Perhaps unbeknownst to you, after being exposed to this sport for some period of time, you've probably been conditioned to believe that serious runners can continually improve only if they spend their hard-earned money on technological solutions–things like expensive heart-rate monitors, sweat-wicking shirts, hydration backpacks, postrun recovery nostrums, electrolyte-coated jelly beans, bionic strength powder, socks designed by NASA, and a fancy GPS watch that gives you your pace down to the 100th decimal point.

An entire cottage industry has risen up around runners. Look at all those sales booths that get in your way as you try to pick up your race bib the day before your big marathon. There they are with their samples, telling you to wear this, to eat this–and most importantly, to *buy* this. If you have it in your hands, if you do as they say, if you read the instructions and pop in three AAA batteries, you'll run faster. Visa and MasterCard accepted; cash preferred, of course. These salespeople hawking quick fixes to complex problems are as old as snake oil itself.

But what no one bothers to say or write about running is that you don't *need* any of this to run faster. Really.

If you want to run faster, you have to realize that you only *need* a few things: your legs, lungs, heart, and a positive attitude. These are the things humans need to make them run faster. Without them, personal records aren't possible. Your legs propel you down the track. Your heart and lungs deliver that precious oxygenated blood to your muscles. A positive attitude contributes to that heroic kick needed to win the race or break that once-elusive personal record.

They matter most.

You have these things on you now. You don't need to buy them in a store; they aren't found by a search engine, so save your time and money. Put down that credit card. Close your browser window. Take a deep breath and prepare yourself to learn about a fresh, worry-free approach to your running.

The intention of this book isn't necessarily to demonize the running industry. After all, what's wrong with well-intentioned people (like this author) trying to make some money? The primary purpose of this book is to give you an alternative to the norm. It's to strike a balance. It's to ground you—something every runner needs. I chose to title this book *Run Simple* because I believe many self-help running books are some variation of the title "Run Complicated." There is something inherently Western about throwing money and technology at problems. In running, this means expecting these store-bought extras will help make up the difference in skill or ability that separates you from the person who crosses the finish line before you do. Sometimes it is as simple as looking in the wrong places for solutions to problems.

What's really missing, usually, is hard work. Those two words should be repeated in all-caps and shouted from the mountaintops: HARD WORK.

Hard work—painful miles run in freezing temperatures; arduous mile repeats in Mombasa-like dew-point air; grueling, lactic-acid-infusing hill repeats—will make you a better runner. That's right, your running improvement is not a mystery waiting to be solved by someone else. You won't necessarily run faster because you are wearing a GPS watch and know *exactly* how far and fast you're running *all the time*. You won't defeat your archrival thanks solely to that aerodynamic singlet at the next race. I'm skeptical about the efficacy of these things and believe that they compound a runner's worry. They can lead to fitness confusion or analysis paralysis. Your purchase of these nostrums and doohickeys will only help some entrepreneurial inventors somewhere.

Your bank account, not your times, will decrease.

Decreasing your finishing times—getting from one point to another faster than you ever have before—that's what I want to help you accomplish with this book, but I also want you to look at running differently; I want you to look at it as you've never looked at it before.

I hope this book helps you. I hope it becomes dog-eared. I hope you write in its margins. Keep it close by. Consult it often. Take it with you on race day and thumb through it while you wait for the race director to call you to the start line. When you feel compelled to buy a $150 pair of running shoes, when the slick ad promising the big personal record has you reaching for your wallet, when you seek to Web surf your way to a site that boasts rapid improvement, have this book ready by your side as a common-sense defense.

So what makes me uniquely qualified to make this case? Why should you bother reading what I've written? How is this book different than any other running book out there?

Unless you pay attention to the history of relatively obscure worldwide ultramarathon stage race results, or keep on top of American marathon rankings from a few years ago, or check the byline of the most recent elite runner interview, you most likely haven't heard about me. But I do have a story to tell—a compelling story, I believe—that makes a strong case for a return to simple running.

Discovering Simplicity

My adventures with running simple began back in 2002, when I was 30 years old. At that time, admittedly not the best period of my life, I weighed over 230 pounds. I wore large pants with an elastic waistband. My doctor told me the obvious: I was overweight and had high blood pressure. My chin was doubled. My food portions were large. I snacked a lot on candied orange slices and ate too many deep-fried saturated fats. I walked practically nowhere. I had to do something about my health. Faced with this troubling news, I made a commitment to change some things in my life.

In high school, I had been a somewhat successful runner, going under 10:20 for the 2-mile event and coming pretty close to making it to the California State High School Cross-Country Championships in my senior year. I originally discovered running after an abysmal career as a ninth-grade wrestler, during which I knew exactly how many lights there were on the gym ceiling thanks to all the torment inflicted on me. I obviously couldn't wrestle, but I could beat the wiry wrestlers when it was time for the team to go for a run during practice, so I decided to try out for the cross-country team.

That's when I first fell in love with running.

Since then, running has always been a source of peace for me. I frequently turn to it as a way to cope with various crises, and so in 2002, when I was at my heaviest, I donned a pair of trainers and signed up for my first marathon.

Struggling a bit financially at the time, I was unable to afford another pair of shoes after my first pair appeared to wear out. I decided to keep running in them as long as possible. They continued to work just fine. I didn't get injured. Despite what other running experts had advised regarding a shoe's lifespan, I was holding up OK on those well-worn pieces of rubber. While wearing that same, tired pair, I logged up to 70-mile weeks of decent marathon training for weeks on end.

Salespeople from the shoe companies probably don't like to read this kind of contrarian writing, but that one battle-hardened pair of shoes with well over 1,000 miles on them managed to keep me injury free and got me to the start of my first marathon in pretty decent shape. I didn't realize it back then, but this lesson in shoe survival was my first introduction to running minimalism.

I ran my first marathon, the Vermont City Marathon, in 3:45, which was good, but not great. Still, by training for it, I was able to lose over 60 pounds. My trusty shoes eventually gave out. A stubborn creature of habit, I bought another pair of the same kind and put another thousand miles on it.

Minimalism gradually took hold in other facets of my running. But I first went through my own phase of throwing money at the problem before I finally gave up on the concept of technology as a running cure-all. Determined to improve on my first marathon time (in an effort to qualify for the Boston Marathon), I bought an enormous, first-generation GPS watch that sat along my forearm like a plastic slug. It rarely worked. I spent more time calibrating the thing and waiting for it to acquire the right number of satellites. I wore it in the rain one too many times, and it broke. It flashed various error codes and then stopped flashing altogether. I also invested in boxes of sports gels and the special fuel-belt contraptions that hold them. I bought technical running shirts and French Foreign Legion-style hats. They worked to some degree, but I just didn't feel comfortable in them. I went to so many race expos and witnessed so many fads that I began to develop a bad taste in my mouth about the whole state of the sport. It all seemed so silly to me.

A discipline as simple and graceful as running, a mostly solitary sport that embraces and values hard work, a free-spirited ritual that takes monk-like focus, patience, and an amazing tolerance for pain and suffering, had been invaded by crass commercialism and lab-coat-wearing entrepreneurs.

In these race expos, I wanted to mount the stage with a giant megaphone and tell everyone that there are no short-cuts. There is only hard work. Put your money away. Walk to the exits and just go running in the clothes you are wearing. Don't buy $30 massage sticks; there are plenty of real sticks out on the trails. Don't get lured into drinking the electrolyte Kool-Aid; cup your hands and drink water from a garden hose while wolfing down chunks of dried pineapple.

And so I began to gradually turn my back on all that. I evolved.

My wintertime running clothes became layers of my old Army gear and holey race T-shirts that I had begun to acquire thanks to entering numerous 5Ks and 10Ks. After shelling out $25 for a pair of fancy gloves and then having my dog bury one of them in an unknown location, I turned to the dollar store as the place to solve my hand-warmth problems. Later that winter, I slipped on a nasty patch of black ice and ripped a $70 pair of sweatpants. My next pair came from Target and cost $29. My watch was basic; on the run it didn't tell me anything other than elapsed time and how fast my splits were. By the end of 2003, after many miles and hard-fought workouts, I had whittled an hour off my marathon personal record, getting my time down to 2:48. And by 2005, after my 16th career marathon, I ran a 2:32 personal record, which translated into a top-300 American time that year.

For a competitive and dedicated male runner in his prime, a 2:32 marathon isn't all that much to brag about. What's important, though, is the philosophical evolution I went through as a runner.

In 2006, I won my first marathon. A year later, I traveled to India and competed in the five-day, 100-Mile Himalayan Stage Race. Going neck-and-neck with a very capable Spanish mountain runner all the way to the race's final stage, I ultimately prevailed. As I trained for these races, I continued to refine my belief that simple and cheap was the way to go.

When I'm not running, I coach and have assisted numerous runners achieve personal bests and qualify for the prestigious Boston Marathon. My athletes' dedication and hard work were the primary reasons for their progress, but I do believe that the concepts I espouse in this book about simple running, which I imparted to them in their training, played some role in their success.

To the Heart of Africa

Enough about me; let's instead examine the current trends in world-class distance running to further substantiate the need for a return to simple running. One glance at the World and Olympic championship medal podiums is enough to realize that technological advancement does not correlate with long-distance-running success. Kenya and Ethiopia, two East African nations with a fraction of the United States' GDP, practically own the sport.

Take for instance the former world-record holder in the marathon, Haile Gebrselassie. Ethiopia's greatest marathoner and arguably one of the best long-distance runners ever ran most of his life with practically nothing. One of 10 children who lived with his family on a farm, Gebrselassie didn't have access to current technology to aid his running. A digital watch was an unaffordable luxury. Specially designed running shoes with computer chips implanted in the insoles were unthinkable. A heart-rate monitor? A GPS watch that gives pace in metric and imperial units? An iPod specifically designed to entertain with special motivational songs during the hard parts of the run?

He had none of these things.

Gebrselassie just ran; he walked, too. As a child, he covered the 10K distance back and forth to his school barefoot (see White, 2011). He didn't take a bus. His parents didn't drive him everywhere. He didn't carry around a smartphone. He ran free of this kind of technology. Gebrselassie is just one example. There are so many more.

In fact, at this very moment, runners all over Africa—poor runners, struggling runners, runners with Olympic medal dreams in their heads—are just going out and simply putting one foot in front of the other over and over again. They run on dusty tracks wearing cheap training sweats and whatever shoes they can find or are given. This subsistence-like living doesn't impede their running; it aids it. These runners aren't burdened with confusing graphs, endless data, and contradicting Web sites.

They don't need any of that nonsense.

So read this book and make a commitment to consider a fresh approach to your running. That's all that matters. I want this book to be more about shifting your attitude than about gleaning specific training tidbits. I would like you to fundamentally change how you approach your running and be conscious of the external forces that seek to influence you and use you to make a profit. More importantly, however, I hope reading this book makes you a faster, happier runner.

Congratulations on taking the first step toward simplifying your running, and good luck.

two

Turn It Off and Tune It Out

So what's wrong with relying on running gadgetry? And how can it prevent you from becoming a better runner?

Here are but a few reasons:

Running Gadgets Waste Your Time

Think about what goes into acquiring and using a GPS watch. First, you have to shop for the right watch. But what exactly is the right watch for you? How do you know what you need from a device that will tell you exactly where you are at all times, how fast and far you are running, as well as how may meters of elevation you climbed and descended? Do you want a watch that connects to the Web? Do you want a watch with an extra-large display? Do you want a night-friendly watch? Which is the best watch for cold climates? Does the cold-climate-friendly watch perform well in the heat? Which watch allows you to Facebook while you are running? How about Twitter? Can you Tweet and Facebook with it? What does *Consumer Reports* have to say about all these things? Which watch does your running buddy recommend?

Researching what the best device is for you takes time. After all, a nice GPS watch isn't a small-ticket item. When you buy one you are making a significant investment, so due diligence is required.

Assuming, then, that you've found the right watch and have made the purchase, just what are you going to do with all the information that the device collects and reports? After your run, you can download everything to your computer. But first, don't forget, you have to install the watch software and then read how to use the watch software. That completed, you are then free to analyze everything! You can graph your average pace over a month, find out exactly how many miles you ran in a week, and determine the average amount of elevation gained or lost. You can summon the power of your computer's brilliant microprocessor to slice and dice all this data into impressive-looking charts and graphs.

Alternatively, you could save hours if not days of your time by strengthening your legs, lungs, and mind by using this time to simply go out and run, but that's boring and tedious, right?

Running Gadgets Are Distractions

In order to use most heart-rate monitors, a runner has to don an uncomfortable plastic strap that senses the heart's pounding and transmits that vital information to a watch. Wear this constrictive thing on a hot day and you will find yourself continually fidgeting with it as it slides down your chest. And what happens when the sensor doesn't work or is blocked by your body? What happens when it gets too wet? In most cases, your heart-rate monitor will beep at you, telling you that something is wrong. This forces you to do one of two things: ignore it, or stop running and fix the problem. Both options stink. Distracting beeping noises don't allow your mind to focus on the run, while stopping a run to adjust a strap or silence that annoying monitor can completely interrupt a workout.

however, are quite capable of gauging these metrics on their own. You are much more reliable for pace and distance calculation than a device that depends on a clear line of sight to orbiting tracking satellites. Why not learn how to use what you already have on you instead of shelling out your hard-earned money to buy a less reliable gadget?

The Web Contains Contradictory Information

The next time you are at a computer, pull up a browser window and search for the term "marathon training." Thirty-seven million results later, you are presented with quite a panoply of "how to run your goal time" suggestions that includes everything from logging a paltry 26 miles a week to full-time professional athlete schedules that entail 140 miles, an oxygen tent, and a special weight-lifting machine. Some sites will tell you to walk during the marathon, while others frown on (and mock) the practice. How far should you run in training before you take on a marathon? The ranges of opinion on the Web are as diverse as the stars in the universe. After searching for the "right" answer to your query, you will most likely conclude what most runners conclude about training advice: it depends.

To add insult to injury, there seems to be a medical study published every day that leads runners to draw various conflicting conclusions about their training. Is carbohydrate loading before a marathon worthwhile? One study says yes, while another says no. Is barefoot running good for you? One evolutionary scientist will wholeheartedly agree, while one podiatrist will tell you it's a recipe for a stress fracture.

It's you, the runner, who is left scratching your head. It's up to you to decide who's correct based on the most compelling argument or research study.

Who has the right answers?

"It depends."

It always depends.

Constantly Surfing the Web in Search of Improvement Can be a Waste of Time

Give or take a few hundred thousand results, a simple Google search on the term "running" yields approximately 1.8 billion Web-page results. Where to start? While it's true that the Web can be incredibly informative and useful, it's also true that it can lead a passionate, overzealous runner into a confused state of information overload. This book doesn't argue for you to abstain from the Internet. This book isn't about becoming a diehard Luddite or completely ignoring science and exercise physiology; it's not called *Run, Simpleton.* We all use the Web; it's a great resource. Just take it down a notch. Don't waste your time Googling all day. If you can't figure something out through the Web about your running, give it a rest for a while. Do something else.

How about going for a run?

Isn't Your Life Already Complex Enough?

In any one day, each of us could be engaging in one or more of the following virtual activities: emailing, Blackberry-checking, iPhone-talking, iPad-typing, Twittering, Facebooking, texting, and Web browsing. Don't you agree that things are getting a little out of hand? We are constantly bombarded with tons of information. Our attention spans are shortening. We must multitask to survive. Type-A behavior is the rule. Do you have any one part of your day where you are actually free from all this flashing madness? Do you ever get any time to yourself to be in complete silence?

Time to Find the "Off" Button and Lock It All Up

After you finish this chapter, please put the book down and go collect all the electronic devices that you run with—all the cords and various installation CDs, too. Financial experts advise people with credit-card-addiction problems to take their cards, dip them in a tub of water, and stick them in the freezer. If they really need to use a card, they will have to wait for them to thaw. I can't tell you to do that with your heart-rate monitor, but I do want you to do something similar.

Lock everything up in a large box and give the key to someone you trust—someone who believes in you and wants you to run faster and with less worry. A good, trusting person for this key would be someone who is exposed to your frequent running complaints and might be frustrated hearing them all the time. Tell this person what you are doing and why you are giving them this strange key. When you feel the need to listen to your music or find out, thanks to orbiting satellites with minimal cloud cover, exactly how fast you are running *all the time*; when you feel the need to ignore your own internal pace clock—then you must ask for the key.

But before you get that key back, you have to agree on certain things with this person. Maybe you agree that you will first reread this book. Maybe you have to run for 90 minutes before you get it back. Maybe you have to go to a race or a local track and watch elite Africans train—Africans who seem to not need all these silly contraptions that you have locked up and are requesting back.

Whatever it is, make it hard to return to your former complex running life. Keep it off and keep it far away from you.

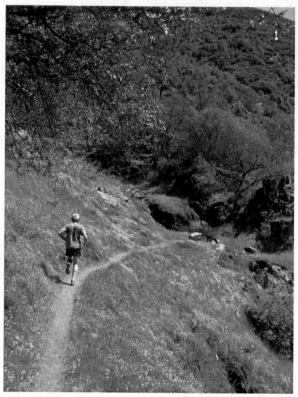

Most of the time, you need to get out there and "just run."
(*Meghan Hicks*)

Three Concepts

NOW THAT YOU ARE FREE FROM THE TECHNOLOGICAL YOKE, it's time to learn how to run simple. But first, pick up any other running book. Thumb through it until you see the training schedules; almost all these types of books have them. They're usually toward the back. Most of these books contain tables with numbers expressed in weekly mileage, time, percentage run at goal pace, time spent at lactate threshold pace, maximum heart rate reserve, target heart rate, or some other convention that requires quite a bit of knowledge about exercise physiology to decipher. These books can do two things to runners: confuse them and make them worry.

The worrying part is what does all the damage.

After tearing out these schedules and taping them to the wall in front of their treadmills, serious runners will usually try to follow them to a T. They will use the book-supplied formulas to figure out exactly how fast they should be running each day. Overwhelmed by science-book-sounding terms like "anaerobic threshold," "resting heart rate," "VO2 max," "VDOT," "glycogen depletion," "oxygen debt," and "lactic acid," runners will then set out and try to do exactly what the book tells them to do. If they can't run as fast or as far as the formula prescribes, they immediately begin to worry. If their biofeedback isn't as it should be, doubt creeps in. Training runs become supreme stress festivals. Workouts turn into big tests—do-or-die evaluations that can be worse than a college-entrance exam. Ulcers form. Nails are bitten, fingers chewed, sleep lost. By the time race day arrives, these poor runners have become their own worst enemies.

A formula doesn't make the runner.

Professional Consistency

One of the most successful elite women's coaches, Ray Treacy, says there is no secret to his athletes' success. What matters most, he says, is training consistency. Treacy maintains that his athlete Molly Huddle was able to break the American outdoor 5,000-meter record in 2010 by putting in workouts without injury interruption. (Larkin 2010a)

Running well doesn't come from checking off a precise list of perfectly executed workouts and sufficiently long runs. Achieving a personal record isn't going to happen because you balanced an equation. It comes from consistently running smart and staying injury-free as long as possible. If you can run as much as possible, if you can maximize your effort on your hard days and your recovery on your easy days, if you can run with as little worry and as much confidence as possible, your faster times will come.

Trust me; they will.

What it means to run simple can be boiled down to three concepts: "Race," "Just Run," and "Rest." All the schedules you will refer to in this book tie in to these concepts. You'll no longer need your heart-rate monitor. You can take your GPS watch back to the sporting-goods store. And on some days, your Rest days, you won't even be wearing a watch. A pair of running shoes, a basic watch, and some positive motivation is what you need most. Before diving into what to do on what day, let's first get to the bottom of what it means to Race, Just Run, and Rest.

Every training day in this book serves some distinct purpose. You shouldn't look at every day as an opportunity to run as fast or as far as possible. Every day isn't an evaluation to see if the hard work you've put in is paying off. You won't get better if you don't allow your body time to recover after it's worked hard. Like everything else in life, your training should be balanced.

Remember this.

If you are running on a Rest day, then you should be recovering from your last run—not stressing or pushing yourself. If it's your day to Race, then give 100 percent. And don't forget that your "100 percent" can change day to day. You won't always run as strong as possible every single Race day. You can't expect all your hard sessions to get better as you progress throughout your schedule. You aren't a robot that can be calibrated; you're human. You wake up stronger on some days than you do on others. You have a lot of other responsibilities in your life, and they can and will affect your performance.

Between these harder Race days and your easy Rest days are what I call your Just Run days.

Specifically, each day serves the following purpose:

Race

These are your hard days. You run harder on these days than on the other two days. Typically, you will Race two or three days a week. On these days, you will be running at paces faster than your goal race pace. These race workouts build strength and are designed to give you confidence.

Not every Race day will be equal in terms of distance covered or time elapsed. Some days may be harder or longer in duration than others. But the key is the word "Race." When you are racing, you are taking the body into new territories. You are asking more of it than it probably wants to give you. Like a car that is suddenly stressed when the driver pushes the gas pedal to the floor, so, too, will your body be stressed. Be on guard for injury on these days. Since these types of workouts demand the most of you, mentally and physically, they are interspersed in the schedules with the optimum amount of Rest days in between. The key is to come into your Race day fresh and rested—primed to run fast.

Pacing on your Race days will vary, depending on the type of workout you are completing, and in keeping with the run simple nature of this book, there will be days of the schedule where I suggest you not even wear a watch.

Why is this?

I believe the need for instant pace feedback can handicap runners and get them overly dependent on external sources. Your body comes with an internal pace clock. Not many runners use it.

I want you to.

Just Run

These are your foundational days. Just Run days usually involve longer distances and more time than your other days. Their purpose is primarily to strengthen muscles, tendons, and ligaments in your legs and feet, and get your body used to consistent running. There are usually three Just Run workouts in a seven-day week. On these days, you are running at paces between your Rest and your Race days.

Rest

The only purpose these runs serve is to give your body whatever it needs to recover after it's worked hard. Rest runs promote the flow of blood throughout the body and facilitate the elimination of waste that has built up in your muscle tissue during workouts run at paces faster than your goal race pace. On Rest days you will also focus on the mental relaxation and think positively about your upcoming workouts and races. In a seven-day week, there are usually two Rest days, but that number can change depending on various factors. For the most part, you won't be wearing a watch on these days. And occasionally you won't even be running on your Rest day. No matter what, you have to take it easy on these days. You have to stay disciplined and fight the urge to overachieve, because pushing your body too much deprives it of the break it rightly deserves and needs.

Goal Race	Advanced	Intermediate	Beginner
Marathon	<3:10 men/<3:29 women	3:10-3:59 men/3:30-4:20 women	Just finish it
Half Marathon	<1:30 men / <1:39 women	1:31-1:53 men / 1:40-2:03 women	Just finish it
10K/5K (5K goal)	<19:00 men / 21:00 women	20:00-25:00 men / 22:00-27:00 women	Just finish it

Training Schedules Explained

This book provides three sample schedules to study based on your ultimate racing goal—a marathon (16 weeks), a half marathon (12 weeks), or a 5K/10K (8 weeks)—and your desired finishing time, broken out as follows:

Keep in mind that these guidelines are rough estimates of performance. Don't get fixated on (or defensive about) these labels. You may have been completing marathons 10 years ago but took a long break and want to get back into them. Accordingly, your first goal back is to just finish the marathon. Does that make you a beginner?

Absolutely not.

One word of caution in selecting which schedule to study: be realistic with your goals. If you've never run a marathon, but, based on your finishing times in previous races at a shorter distance, you think you are an advanced marathoner, I would still advise you to examine the intermediate schedule at the beginning. If you find it too easy or not challenging enough after the first few weeks, transition to the advanced schedule. Better to err on the side of caution than get hurt or immediately soured by the marathon training experience.

So, before determining which schedule you are most interested in studying, examine all the schedules in detail. You will notice that they differ in the following areas:

Number of repetitions during your "Race" days. The harder the schedule, the more repetitions you are usually doing. I designed the schedules this way because I'm assuming the seasoned runner is heading into the schedule already accustomed to workouts like these.

Time spent running. The more advanced the runner, the more time on the feet I prescribe during your Rest and Just Run days. This assumes that a more capable runner can handle more volume, and, in order to run faster, will need more of an opportunity to build up general length strength and increase efficiency. Someone whose goal is to just finish his first race doesn't need to overachieve here.

Recovery time on Race days. The suggested duration you rest between your track workouts on your Race days is reduced for the more advanced runners because they tend to run their repetitions faster than someone of lesser ability.

Types of recovery. Walking is part of the Beginner and Intermediate plans, but not the Advanced plan. That being said, there's nothing wrong with an Advanced runner choosing to walk occasionally on a Rest day.

All in a Day's Purpose

As stated earlier, each day of the schedule assigns you a specific purpose (i.e., Race, Just Run, or Rest). Within each type of day, there are several distinct types of workouts you will complete. Each type of workout focuses on different components of your running.

Rest Runs

There are five "Rest" runs in the sample schedules: "No Watch," "Green," "Mind," "Walk," and "Day Off," Regardless of what your purpose is on any given Rest day, make sure you are taking it easy. If you are breathing hard (physical stress) or worrying (mental stress) you aren't resting.

It is important to maximize down time on your Rest days. This means more than just taking it easy beforehand. Most runners preparing for a big workout the next day try to get a good night's sleep. This is great, but also try to get as much sleep as possible before any of your "Rest" days. After your "Rest" run, also try to take it easy. You should internalize that concept all day. Try not to do any other hard physical activity on your rest days. Paint the house and mow the lawn on a different day if possible.

No Watch. Don't wear a watch on these days. Run a familiar course that would take you approximately 40 to 45 minutes to complete if you ran it as easily as possible. If you are a first-time runner who doesn't have a well-known course at the tip of your fingers, time a few of your planned No Watch routes at an extremely relaxed pace so that you have a starting point for future No Watch days. Don't stress about the time or the distance. No Watch means exactly that: no watch. It doesn't mean wear a watch and don't look at it. Leave the thing at home. On days that you are to be recovering, you shouldn't be spending any effort to measure how long you are running. Your pace should be extremely relaxed—to the point that you almost feel like you should be running faster. No Watch days are meant to be welcome breaks from hard and long running. They should be completely enjoyable runs free of worry. If you run with someone, explain to your partner what you are doing and ask that he or she kindly not wear a watch.

If your partner is edging ahead of you during a No Watch run, resist the urge to catch up. Ask him to slow down, and remind him that you are taking it easy today. Quite often, groups of competitive people who run together on an easy day end up racing at the end as each runner unthinkingly ratchets up the pace. Jumping in with a group of superfast runners who like to do this can be an excellent idea on your Race or Just Run days, but avoid doing so on your Rest days.

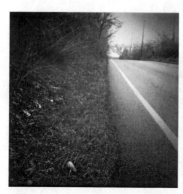

There are plenty of opportunities to clean up your running space on a "Green" run. (*Author*)

Green. On this Rest day, bring an empty trash bag (or bags) with you (and a pair of rubber gloves if you want) and pick up garbage you see along your running route. Your goal is to try to fill the bag(s) during your run. You don't have to hurry while you pick up trash, because this is a Rest run. Pace and time aren't a factor. Doing something praiseworthy for the environment while working the legs and lungs at a leisurely pace is the name of the game here. A Green run isn't meant to be on-the-run garbage collection. Instead, feel free to stop long enough to pick it up. If carrying a large bag of smelly trash doesn't sound like jolly-good-times fun to you, then plan to drop the bags off on the side of the road as you fill them and collect them later. You could also coordinate with your town or city beforehand. Tell them what you plan on doing. They might give you specially marked bags and may even offer to do the bag pickup for you.

Many companies and other organizations sponsor miles for garbage collection. Think about your Green run as a one-person sponsorship. Make it a goal to keep your mile or miles as free of trash as possible. And you might be surprised to find that your actions influence other runners to do the same.

Understandably, bending over and picking up trash can be asking a lot of you. Roadside garbage is downright disgusting. So don't feel bad discriminating in what you decide to collect. You don't have to pick up everything. One possibility is to look for empty soda cans, or maybe make a rule that you will only pick up recyclables. If you

Help Put Others Back on Their Feet
If you live near a large U.S. city, find out if the Back on My
Feet charity has a presence there. Back on My Feet is an out-
standing homeless-outreach program that promotes self-suffi-
ciency through running. It is always looking for eager volunteer runners like you, and volunteering there may be a great
way to complete your "Green" runs.

get money for recycling bottles and cans in your state,
donate the proceeds to a charity of your choice. The fact
that you are taking some sort of positive steps to improve
the environment is to be applauded As you start to do
more of these Green runs, hopefully you will begin to see
that you are making a positive difference in some way.
Taking those kinds of selfless actions can be a perfect salve
for days when you may not be feeling your best physically
and mentally. You may have just bombed your workout
the day before or had a hard time keeping up with a group
that was running your goal pace. You may be questioning
a lot of things; your confidence may be flagging. But as you
begin to do something concrete like making the space you
play in every day more beautiful, you will begin to recover
and hopefully regain any lost confidence in your abilities.

If you aren't down with garbage collection and the dirt
that goes with it, there are plenty of alternatives for your
Green run. Come up with your own. The gist is to do
something for someone or something. Make the run about
anything other than yourself. Selflessness is a healthy
notion that can promote recovery. You could use the run
to greet or encourage fellow runners or any like-minded
exercise enthusiasts. Alternately, you could spend the run
planning a selfless task like volunteering at a race, a home-
less shelter, or a soup kitchen. It could be doing something
nice closer to home, like planning out a delicious meal that
you will cook for your family that night.

Whatever you do, make it all about someone or something else that day. So much of running is about you and

your goals; take a moment to put others first on this day. In the end, it may help you become not only a better runner, but also a better person.

Mind. On these Rest runs, spend the whole time visualizing success in achieving your racing goals. Think about setting that personal record. As you get closer to race day, imagine yourself running the course. Imagine all those race-pace miles feeling good. Create images in your head of how you want the race to unfold. Tell yourself that it will be that way—over and over again. If you are trying to qualify for the Boston Marathon, think about what it will feel like when you ultimately toe the line in Hopkinton—how elated you will feel to have done something so few are capable of doing. During these runs, also be thankful for being able to run, regardless of finishing time. Be thankful that you are healthy enough to put one foot in front of the other. Think about all the good things going on in your life. Sure, you have your challenges and setbacks. We all have these. But on this run, these negative thoughts should be crowded out of your head. Only positive thoughts are allowed on the run. Finish the run happy to be alive. If you are wearing a watch, try not to consult it except for hitting the start button at the beginning and the stop button at the end. And since this is a "Rest" run, time and pace are immaterial.

Other than just taking it easy and thinking positively on these days, consider changing a few things to help you recover. So much is written in running books about how to run hard, but so very little is written about how to run easy. Most serious runners are driven like mad. They know they need to run hard on workout days and push the pace, but what does it really mean to recover? The majority of running coaches will tell their athletes to "take it easy" and "rest up" for the next onslaught coming their way in two days. It's usually phrased in terms of the difficulties that lie ahead in the training week, and so little is said about the Rest day itself.

Rest Like a Pro
He represented the United States in the 5,000-meter run at the 2004 Olympics. Now Tim Broe coaches runners. One of the biggest lessons he learned as an athlete that he's trying to impart is how to relax between training sessions. "My biggest thing was to learn to calm down and just relax during the day. I couldn't just train in the morning, sit around all day, and then train at night," he says. "I want [my athletes] to try and relax and not do so much throughout the day. I used to work out in the morning, golf in the afternoon, run around for the rest of the day, and then just be exhausted at night." (Larkin 2010b).

Here are some ideas to try out that will help you properly rest:

Watch the sun rise. On one of your Mind days, try to get up before daybreak and head out on the roads or trails at the moment the sun starts to rise. Try to find a locale where you can see as much of the horizon as possible. Watching a sunrise can be an incredibly energizing and moving experience.

Enjoy a moon run. Plan one of your Mind runs at night when there is a full moon and clear skies. Get out of areas with light pollution, and when you are running, take a look up at the magnificence of the stars and planets over your head. Check the news for periods with meteor showers and try to do your run in the middle of them. Another way to experience a fun nighttime Mind run is to study the constellations and stargaze on the run.

Always seek nature. The less distraction, the easier it is to be at peace with yourself. Make your Mind runs as nature-filled as possible. Run by a body of water like a large lake, or cruise the trails along a ridgeline. Go rural. Stay off the roads. Avoid cars and other noise pollution. Silence is what you seek.

Start your Mind run the right way. Try to find about 5 to 10 minutes of quiet before your run. Don't just don your trainers and rush out the door. Sit on your front porch or go for a brief contemplative walk before you start your run. You want to set the right tone. We are rushing so much all day that we

forget to properly transition from office meetings, buzzing cell phones, and Facebook/Twitter updates into a period of calmness and peace.

Complement the run with a good book or an inspirational movie. You can't go wrong with *Chariots of Fire* or John L. Parker's classic novel, *Once a Runner.* Treat yourself to something relaxing or motivating on your "Mind" days.

Walk. This Rest activity is prevalent in the beginning and intermediate schedules. Walk for the prescribed amount of time. Ambling is fine. Admire the scenery. You don't have to put your head down and "race walk," moving your arms as fast as possible. Walking is a fantastic way to exercise. It promotes circulation, burns calories, and builds leg strength.

Walking definitely isn't for wimps. The Finns of the 1920s were the Kenyans of today. Back then they dominated long-distance running and caused the sporting world to gape, open-mouthed in wonder and amazement, at their feats. Paavo Nurmi, "The Flying Finn," led the way for them with an astounding 20 world records. He also secured gold medals in the 10,000-meter track, 10,000-meter cross-country, and 10,000-meter team cross-country events of the 1920 Olympics. The Finns rounded out their domination of the distance events in those Olympics with Hannes Kolehmainen's marathon victory. The Finnish running code was ultimately deciphered in a book written by J. J. Mikkola in 1929 (see Noakes, 1991).

What was their secret? GPS? Heart-rate monitors? Rigorous, meticulous schedules using abaci and alchemy? High-altitude houses?

Walking.

The Finns walked as part of their training during the brutal Nordic winters. Marathoners would do anywhere from 10 to 20 miles of walking from December to March. The last parts of the walks (2 to 6 miles) were run. As spring approached, walking was phased out and more running phased in (see Noakes, 1991).

Keep in mind that unlike other coaches out there, I'm not suggesting that you walk in the middle of a race or that you walk on a Race day. Walking is purely part of recovery. It's to be done on your Rest day.

Keep in mind, too, that walking isn't limited to the Walk days on this schedule. Please walk as much as possible. If you spend most of your time at work sitting in a cubicle or office, then make it a habit to take walk breaks of 10 to 15 minutes once an hour. For some jobs this may not be possible, so just do what you can. Walk when the opportunity presents itself. Park far away from the office door and take the stairs instead of the elevator. Any time you sit in front of the steering wheel of your car, ask yourself this question: can I walk there?

Don't spend your time finding excuses why you can't walk somewhere; find the ways to get it done, and make it happen. If your grocery store is down the road, don't say you can't walk there because you need a car to transport your groceries. Borrow your child's wagon or carry a rucksack. Every little bit of walking helps runners of all abilities. Walking isn't just for slower, overweight runners.

If walking takes too long and you don't have the time to incorporate more of it into your life, then ride a bike. Get a basket or a trailer for it so you can use it to transport things.

The key here is to get the heart rate up and get the legs moving. It's an attitude shift. Look at every little bit of exercise and activity you do as a way to help your overall running health.

Day Off. A day off is a day off—it's not anything else. This option is not negotiable and is primarily incorporated in the Beginner plans to allow newer runners with less developed muscles and lungs more time to rest and recover. Don't cheat on your days off by sneaking in "just" 30 minutes of easy running. You are encouraged to stay active, but you shouldn't be doing anything that's making you sweat on these days. Cut yourself some slack.

Rest > Just Run > Race

Just Run Days

This concept is called Just Run because on these days, just getting out and running is your primary focus. You aren't worrying about pace like you are on your Race and Rest days. You are doing a lot of the same thing on these days. Repetition is an absolutely vital component of running. The runner's body has to learn how to adapt to the repeat pounding. On these days you are bridging the gap between your recovery and your racing.

On some days you will be running closer to the Rest line. This can mean a more relaxed-pace run with a few Race-type surges thrown in at the end. Conversely, you may find yourself working pretty hard on your Just Run days. An example of this would be a progression run where you are taking it out really easy and then cranking up the pace gradually until you are going all out at the end. But don't forget that the key component of this training phase is to "Just Run."

You don't really have to "nail" anything. You don't have to be meticulously checking your watch. Other than accomplishing the assigned objective, let go of the steering wheel on these days. Focus on just getting in the miles. Those miles are doing something for you. They are slowly making you more efficient and stronger.

During your Just Run days, you'll complete four workouts: "Hidden Hills," "Progression," "Surges," and "Long Runs."

Specifically, here's what each Just Run workout entails:

Hidden Hills. Surprises in training are essential for any runner. They simulate the chaos of a race, and they can also serve to break up a run's monotony. One way to toss the element of surprise into your training is to randomize your route.

You have two missions to complete on your Hidden Hills days: The first is to find new running routes that you can use later in your training. The second is to sprint up any hill you find while out exploring. No matter your conditioning, you should be winded at the end of this surprise hill sprint. Take it nice and easy on the downhill sections as a way to recover. In the event you are struggling to find new run options for Hidden Hills workouts, then complete any of your standard loops in reverse.

If you are still out of options, then just run your same routes and hammer the hills you already know about. However, no matter where you live, there are most likely numerous places to run that you haven't been to yet, so get out and do some exploring.

Progression. World-class Kenyans love these types of runs. They are an excellent (and safe) way to cover a wide range of paces in one session. Here's how you complete a progression run: Start your run very slow–practically walking. As your run progresses, pick up your pace. Break the progression run into thirds, so the first third is extremely slow, the second third is at a medium pace, and the last third is as fast as possible. Finish your progression run out of breath, as if you were finishing a race. Unlike a track repeat or a tempo workout, progression runs allow the body to gradually ease into an uncomfortable realm. That's why they are a great alternative to harder, more explosive workouts. Another bonus to doing these is that you get to learn how to control your effort. If you go out too fast in the beginning and don't truly pace yourself, you may find yourself doing a progression run in reverse. So if you've never done these before, go easy at first. If you want to, set the timer on your watch to count down the time it takes to do one-third of the run. When the watch beeps, it's time to crank up the pace.

Surges. A surge is a sudden injection of intense pace in the middle or end of an otherwise slower run. Being able to find the mental and physical reserves to surge in the middle of a race is key to countering a possible move by your race-day opponent or making your own move when the time is right. It's also important to be able to surge in the event you find yourself off your goal pace in a race and want to get back on track. The way to complete a surge is to pick up the pace substantially and hold it for the period of time called for in the schedule. Think of surges as shock-to-the-system sprints in the middle (or end) of otherwise leisurely runs. As with anything sudden done to the body when running, be careful with these things. Every time you surge, you stand a chance of doing something harmful, like pulling a muscle or even tripping. Make sure you are sufficiently warmed up before you complete your first surge, and if you feel any sort of acute pain, immediately back off. The pace on your Surge days should otherwise be somewhat relaxed. You aren't taking it too easy, but you also aren't hammering either. Your breathing should come naturally, and your attitude should be such that you feel you could hold your pace with no problems for the duration of the workout. After your surge is completed, don't stop running. Slowing down for a few seconds to catch your breath is OK.

Long Runs. Long Runs are essential components of the distance runner. Some coaches, like the great Arthur Lydiard, swore by them even for his middle-distance athletes, like the 1960 and 1964 Olympic gold medalist in the 800 meters, Peter Snell, who ran 22 miles in New Zealand's Waitakere Ranges. (see Ferstle, 2012)

Why are long training runs so important?

Adaptation.

A long run usually lasts 90 minutes or more. Long runs strengthen muscles and tendons in your legs—your bones, too. They can also increase the size of your capillaries. Larger capillaries mean more oxygenated blood can be delivered to your muscles. Think of the long run as a vital adaptive component of your running. The longer you run, the more efficient your body becomes. If you are training for the half marathon and marathon, longs run are also a great chance to practice for your big race. Consider them dry runs. You should use your long runs to learn and experiment with things like hydration, fueling, and what to wear or not wear.

If you are completing the Advanced schedules, you will be doing some extremely long runs, but they build gradually over time. Your pace for these runs is immaterial unless Surges are specifically called for. Just get it done, and don't get caught up in how fast you are going. Remember when you're out running long that the more time on your feet you get, the stronger you are becoming. Also feel free to experiment with pace progression during your long runs. It's OK to start them extremely slow and build up to a quicker pace at the end.

Race Runs

There are six Race workouts for you to incorporate into your training schedule: "Track Repeats," "End Hills," "Tempos," "Goal Pace," "Tee-to-Green," and "Tune-up" Races. Recall that a Race workout means you will be running at paces faster and longer than when you are completing Just Run and Rest runs.

Track Repeats. If you've been running for a while, then you're surely no stranger to working out on a track. If you've never done these things, then prepare yourself. Barring the race itself and perhaps a longer Tempo run, track workouts are probably the hardest things you will encounter on your running journey.

They take courage and perseverance.

They are invariably run when it's either blazing hot out or in the middle of a tempest. They make you really hurt and sometimes force you to question just what it is you are doing with yourself. But fear not, because they make you a better runner. And when you finish them, you are usually completely spent, but happy to be alive.

They are a rite of passage for all runners.

In this book, all track workouts are given in terms of number of repetitions and recovery time. Specifically, here's how to run your track workouts:

"Recovery" is how much time you have to rest between your repetitions. This is your time, so you can do whatever you want while you rest. Put your hands on your hips. Pour some water over your head. Stay moving if you can. Slowly jog if possible.

Your effort for these sessions should be all-out. Hurl yourself down that track. Push it. Take no prisoners. At the end of the repetition you should be breathing hard and may find yourself bent over with your hands on your knees, panting, and staring at pebbles and ants on the ground.

Go ahead and time the repetitions, but don't get caught up running them in a specific time. This "go as fast as you can" guidance deviates from a lot of running books, which usually spell out exactly how fast you should be running your track workouts. There is a time and a place for pace specificity in your workouts. For example, it's important to pay attention to exact pace during some of your goal-pace workouts, but for your track repetitions, just go out and give it your best shot.

Consistency, effort-wise, across all repetitions is desired. That's the goal: allocate your effort evenly. Along these lines, try to imagine that you have only so much energy at the beginning of a track workout. If you are doing four repetitions, then imagine dividing that energy and effort such that each repetition gets exactly one-fourth of your reserves—no more and no less. Don't take it easy in the first three reps and then hammer the last one.

You need to learn how to control your pace. This isn't easy. World-class runners struggle with this, so don't feel bad if you struggle with it as well. Have low expectations going into your schedule's first few track workouts. After you've finished them, think about what went well and what didn't go well. Apply those lessons learned in your subsequent track workouts. Eventually, you should be pretty good at dialing into the pace you need to be at to complete the workout.

Have Realistic Workout Expectations
Coach Tim Broe tries to teach his athletes to manage their expectations when they are working hard on the track. "There are so many guys who are so anxious to get better, they keep pushing and pushing. . . . You do have to push yourself to a certain point, but sometimes you have to let it come to you, too. You've got to learn to relax." (Larkin 2010b)

You know you have run your repetition hard and at the correct pace if you feel some fatigue when it's time to start your next repetition. Nobody ever feels like they get enough recovery between repetitions; that's the point. Consider this: how much recovery time do you get between miles in a race? Zero. You get no breaks in a race, so get used to not getting much in practice. Your body should be pleading for more time to rest. If it's not, then you need to either be running faster or giving yourself less rest.

Don't forget to warm up before your work out. Typically, this entails no less than 20 minutes of easy jogging. Try to find a track that's 20 to 30 minutes' running distance from your home.

Also don't forget to do a cool down afterward. You don't need to immediately start running after you've completed the workout. Give yourself some time to contemplate (and celebrate) what you just did. Pulling off something like a hard 6 x 1,600 meters with a 6-minute rest is no small feat. You deserve to pause, maybe sit on a bleacher, and appreciate the fact that you successfully got the mind to talk the body into doing nearly impossible things. Take a drink of water. Even walk a few laps around the track, and then do your cool down. Be careful on your cool-down runs; you just put your body through its paces and pushed it to the edge of its capabilities.

End Hills. For these Race days, finish your run on a long stretch of hill. Long can be a relative term, so shoot for anything that takes you more than a minute to ascend.

Steepness isn't as important as length. Finish your run uphill as hard as possible. Give it 100 percent, as if you were fighting for first place against a stubborn opponent. This means at the top of the hill, you should be bent over, hands to knees, and breathing hard. Crank it hard on this hill. Get your legs and lungs burning. This workout's purpose is to teach the body and mind to push hard at the end of a race and to allocate effort correctly. So often, runners burn out early in races. These workouts get you used to having some real finishing speed left so you can take on a late-race challenge thrown at you. In this instance, it's a hill, but in a race, it might be a stubborn competitor you can't shake, or something worse: a 20-mph headwind, a hill, and that stubborn competitor. Bringing along a partner during this workout is a great idea; race that person to the top.

This stimulus is usually thrown in at the end of a tough workout like a Tempo, so it will be especially challenging for you to have enough at the end for an all-out sprint at the top of a hill. Prepare yourself accordingly. Know that this workout will be challenging.

Tempos. The word "tempo" is thrown around a lot in running circles. This book throws it around, too, but what exactly does it mean? I define a Tempo run as an uncomfortably paced, longer effort. In this book's workout schedules, this usually translates into about 25 to 50 minutes of sustained work. You are trying to develop the right mixture of speed and endurance in a Tempo run. For your Tempo days, run the workout as if you were running a 10K race. Just as you aren't fretting about the time of your repetitions in a track workout, so, too, don't fret about how much distance you are covering during a Tempo run. Instead, focus on one thing: your breathing. It should be pained, but manageable. When you set out on a Tempo run, you should be able to mentally grasp the pace. It will probably start to hurt 5 to 10 minutes into the run, but it's not at the level of pain that you experience in a track repetition or at the end of a race.

You shouldn't feel compelled to stop.

Gradually increase the pace of your Tempos at the beginning. Start out fast, but err on the side of going out a bit too slow and ease into your Tempo run. The top priority is to complete the workout. At the end of a Tempo run, you should be significantly out of breath. Your legs and lungs should be spent. You should leave the Tempo workout looking forward to a rest day.

As with a track workout, you need to be warmed up beforehand and to cool down afterward. Take about 30 to 40 minutes before the Tempo to prepare your body for the effort. And after 20 minutes of running, do four to six accelerations at what your expected Tempo pace will be. Make the accelerations approximately 20 seconds each, with about a minute between accelerations. These pre-Tempo accelerations will prepare the mind and body for the faster running it's about to do. After your Tempo is complete, cool down for 30 to 40 minutes of extremely slow running.

State parks with public bike paths are excellent places for Tempo runs. If you don't have something like that where you live, plan out a loop in your neighborhood. Experiment with the time and distance of the loop, such that on longer Tempo days you may run several laps of the loop. Loops for Tempo runs are great because you can establish a home base. When you pass the start/stop point, you can shed clothing or even have a fluid bottle ready for a quick swig on a hot day. You can also do Tempo runs on tracks, but only as a last resort. Instead, try to find a natural setting. Ask the owners of your local running store where the university or high school cross-country teams host their meets or practices. If you can find a grass loop for your Tempos, your knees and legs will thank you.

Goal Pace.

If there's one training concept you *have* to internalize after reading this book, it's "Goal Pace." If I had to boil this book down to a few pages, this would be the section I'd keep.

Goal-paced runs are, by far, the most important workouts you will complete in your training.

How can you be expected to race at a given pace for a sustained period of time if your body has no concept of what it feels like to run that fast? Isn't the primary purpose of running training to prepare the mind and body as much as possible for the rigors of race day?

Don't worry if, at the beginning of your training schedule, your Goal Pace runs are difficult.

They should be.

If they are too easy, then think about adjusting your goals. Most likely, longer Goal Pace runs will even be difficult pulling off well into your plan. At first, your breathing will be pained, but as you become more efficient, it should change to sustainably hard. The more sustainable, the more comfort you feel as you grind it out, the better your confidence should be come race day. Hopefully, as you progress through the schedule, your fitness will improve and these Race days become more like Just Run days. Also think about Goal Pace days as little windows that let you peek at your fitness and potential to achieve your race-day goals.

But they can be deceiving, too, so don't look at Goal Pace runs as end-all-be-all workouts. For example, if you are training for a marathon, you are taking on high weekly mileage, long runs, and taxing Race workouts. Your body is beat down from this onslaught, and so marathon-pace efforts will feel harder than they will when race day arrives and you have rested properly beforehand thanks to the tapering process (which will be explained later in the book). A properly executed taper can do a lot to restore your body and get it into prime race-day shape.

Goal Pace runs are broken out in the schedules as "Goal Pace: Watch" and "Goal Pace: No Watch." The differences in these workouts are as follows:

Goal Pace: Watch. Wear a digital watch during this workout and monitor your splits every mile. As you cross the mile markers, take close mental notes on how you feel. If you are off pace, pick it up or slow it down. You have to nail the pace no matter what. On these days it's OK to refer to your watch. Think of your timekeeping device as a guide that is helping you learn what goal pace should feel like.

Goal Pace: No Watch. Optimally, you will conduct these workouts with someone who can time you during the entire workout. If you can't arrange for that, then wear a watch, but don't look at it until you finish the workout. You may also hit the split button on your watch at each mile marker, but don't consult it until the very end. The purpose of this run is to condition your body to memorize goal pace. The more that pace is ingrained in your head, the better the chances are that come race day, you won't make the classic mistake of getting caught up in the excitement and going out too fast.

Memorization of goal pace—or any pace for that matter—is absolutely imperative.

On days that you are doing Goal Pace: No Watch workouts, do a little postrun introspection. Ask yourself a few questions about the workout:

How close was I to my goal pace in total?

How consistent were my splits?

If I used the lap button to secretly record my splits, how did they look?

What will I do differently next time?

Goal Pace for Beginners. If you are a beginner runner and you just want to finish the race, don't be overly concerned about your goal pace. Still, you will need some initial frame of reference in order to complete the goal-pace workouts in this book. As a starting point, use the following first-timer goal times:

Race	Male	Female
Marathon	4:00	4:30
Half Marathon	2:00	2:30
5K/10K (using 5K time)	25 minutes	30 minutes

In your first few Goal Pace runs, dial in your ultimate goal for the race. If the workouts at your desired goal pace are extremely difficult to complete, then relax your goals. The opposite holds true if you have no problems running at goal pace early in the schedule.

Tee-to-Green

This is a generic name for one of my all-time favorite workouts. Understandably, because of the difficulty getting permission to run on a public golf course and the litigiousness of the present world, it may be hard to complete a true Tee-to-Green workout, but here's how to try:

Visit your local public golf course and sit down with the course marshal. Find out the course's policy on before/after hours use of the course for runners. Assuming it's OK, you complete a "Tee-to-Green" workout by starting at the first hole and running from the tee to the putting green as fast as you can. Once you make it to the hole, walk from that green to the next hole. This is the equivalent of your recovery time after a track repetition. The training schedules in this book specify how many holes you will complete that day. There's no need to wear a watch on these days since the distance from the hole to the next tee determines the recovery time.

Why are these workouts so great? Several reasons:

First, if you can run on a golf course, you are off the asphalt and in a pristine, quiet locale. The golf course's soft turf is the perfect place for a fast, low-impact workout. Second, golf courses are mostly random. Unlike a track that has a fixed distance, a golf course introduces chaos into the workout. Some par three holes may only require you to run 250 yards, while others have you doing over double the distance. This means your paces will have to vary from hole to hole. Finally, the dogleg nature of some holes prevents you from seeing the finish. Not being able to see the end point of your repetition makes it more challenging and more true to how a real race unfolds when the finish line isn't in sight until the end.

Tee-to-Green Alternatives

Champing at the bit to give this workout a try, you now head down to your neighborhood public golf course. But your hopes are dashed when the marshal kicks you out of his golf cart, saying your proposal is the strangest thing he's ever heard in his life. He's got to worry about enforcing rules and replacing fairway divots; he doesn't have time for you and your running.

Now what?

No worries. There are ways to simulate a tee-to-green workout.

The Stick-in-the-Ground Approach. Give this alternative a spin at your local state park or nature preserve–anywhere there are sticks and soft ground. For this workout, you'll need a watch and a number of sticks equal to the number of "holes." During your warm-up, head down the path or trail with sticks in hand. At random intervals between 45 seconds and 3 minutes, place the sticks in the ground in easily visible spots. Then look back to see that you can clearly see them from the trail or path. Alternately, you can make your own reusable sticks for these workouts, wrapping them in blaze orange tape so that even a plane could see them.

The randomness of the interval is up to you, but the key is to introduce chaos into your workout. If you put your first marker down after 45 seconds, put the second one down at 90 seconds, and the third one down at 55 seconds. And to simulate the fact that a golf course sometimes "hides" the finish line, place your sticks after a long turn, or maybe bury one of the sticks a little deeper in the ground so you don't see it until you are right up on it.

In order to simulate the recovery from a hole to the next tee, you can jog/walk for 15 to 20 seconds past the marker and then turn around. When you reach your marker, take off again. Or, you could take the complexity up a notch and mark the stop point of one "hole" and the start point of the next "tee." Whatever you do, clean up after yourself. Pack out what you pack in. Don't leave that once-pristine trail full of brightly colored sticks.

The Landmark Workout. A landmark workout is similar to a stick-in-the-ground workout. But instead of marking your course beforehand, you run a randomized amount of time based on landmarks that appear. A good place to do these is on roads. Set your watch timer to three minutes. Start out on your first "hole," and after 45 seconds of all-out running, begin to look for landmarks ahead of you. They can be anything from a telephone pole to something out of place that catches your eye, like an old-fashioned car parked on the side of the road. Since there's so much trash out there, you can even look for a discarded beer can or a plastic water bottle. Pretty much anything will work. Once you decide on the landmark, don't take your eyes off it, because that's your new finish line.

Stop there.

If you can't find a suitable landmark, stop when your watch beeps after three minutes. Use the same recovery technique prescribed in the stick-in-the-ground workout. And don't forget to mix it up. Vary the amount of time you are running between each landmark.

Resorting to the Track. When all else fails, head to the track for this workout. You can use the infield to put down markers, or you can just vary the workout based on the number of laps you complete for each "hole." If you aren't sure how many laps you should complete, consider writing out the workout beforehand. A good and cheap random-lap generator is a six-sided die. For each "hole" you have to complete, roll one die and write down the number rolled. That number corresponds to the number of laps you will run. Use common sense: if you roll a one three times in a row, reroll the die until you get some variability in the workout. The same goes for rolling a lot of fives or sixes—consistently running over a mile per "hole" exceeds the goal of the shorter workout.

Get Creative. A Tee-to-Green workout is meant to be challenging but fun. I challenge you to come up with your own creative workouts using these concepts of randomness, unknown length, variable speed, and a hidden finish line.

Tune-up Races

For days that a Tune-up race is called for, check your local calendar and find a suitable race. The distance of the race called for is indicated in the sample plan. For marathoners and half marathoners, these races are usually 5Ks in the beginning of the schedule and progress in racing distance. Half marathoners will have a maximum racing distance of 10K, whereas marathoners will have one or two half-marathon tune-ups in their schedule. Those working on the 5K and 10K will have some shorter races like the mile.

Just what is a Tune-up race? It's exactly what it sounds like: a workout designed to adjust the body for race-day conditions. It's your shot to learn everything you need to learn about racing before the actual race day. Some Tune-up races should be run at your ultimate goal pace, while others are run at faster paces (for example, tempo-type efforts). The example training schedules spell out these recommended paces. Besides taking your body up to uncomfortable levels of speed and causing it to understand how to persevere and deal with suffering, think of a Tune-up primarily as a learning experience. Don't stress out about your placing or how well you run compared to others. Your aim isn't to win races or age-group divisions. Remember that Tune-up races take place when your body is already dealing with the fatigue of higher mileage and other workouts during the week. Learn from these races. Remember how your body felt while running at goal pace. Internalize the things you did right, and make a note not to do the things you did wrong.

Thou Shalt Not Overcomplicate Things

A final word about all these concepts: They are *general* guidelines for you to use. What's more important than doing the *exact* workout on the *exact* day is that you internalize the concept of worry-free running. Above all else, remember what the purpose of your run is on that particular day: racing, just running, or resting. If it's a Race day and you feel like pushing it harder or longer than the schedule prescribes, then by all means go for it. But if it's a rest day, don't. Common sense trumps everything. So if you wake up with a slight pain in your knee and the schedule calls for a 90-minute run that day, don't do it. Rest that day–even take a no-running day if you need to. Maybe rest the next day as well. Listen to your body. You won't necessarily lose fitness by making that kind of wise decision with your training. Better to live to fight another day than to crash and burn with a foolish injury.

The Sample Plans

What follows are sample training plans covering three areas: a marathon (16 weeks), a half marathon (12 weeks), and a 5K/10K (8 weeks). *Remember that these are sample plans. Change them after you have read this book.* Unless you are new to running, don't follow them exactly. Every runner is unique. Every runner has his own schedule and his own needs. And most likely, every runner who reads this book is going to interpret them differently. Hopefully, everyone will get something from it. Some of you will reject most of it and take one or two things with you. Some of you may take all of it. Some might just walk away with their own ideas for how to simplify their running. This would be great news across the board.

Think of this book as an instruction manual for anatomical pencil drawing. Such a book teaches you technique and is filled with examples of how to draw, for instance, the face of an old man, or the hands of a young woman. If you read that book, you wouldn't think it was designed to teach you how to trace the pictures. Instead, you are consulting it because it teaches you methods and techniques. It provides the pictures as examples, but that old man's face contorts; the young woman's hands move–which makes tracing only

Beware of the Cookie Cutter
Terrence Mahon, coach of the American record-holder in the marathon, Deena Kastor, is wary of fixed training schedules. "I have to say that I have never been a fan of the cookie-cutter approach," he says. "I've always had trouble even as an athlete where you read some guy's training plan in a magazine and say, 'Oh well this must be the be-all-end-all approach.' In reality, you don't know everything that is behind it." (Larkin 2009d)

so good. If you can learn to master the technique, you can draw your own pictures in any circumstance.

Similarly, take these schedules and study them at first, but as your situation changes, as you deal with obstacles like injury and work-life balance, this quaint schedule won't be worth the paper it's printed on. No coaches worth their salt write out 16 long weeks of training not knowing anything about their athletes. They get to know them well. They find out what motivates them and what doesn't motivate them. They understand their performance gaps and seek to fill them in where necessary with the right kind of training. When it's time for a coach to write out a schedule, it's done with a pencil, because the runner's body and mind are in a constant state of flux.

When first setting out to write this book, I was hesitant to include sample training plans for fear that people would look at them as formulas to follow and that they would get wrapped up in the details and obsessed with completing them precisely as written. You can't find exactly what to do with your running by examining one book, let alone 50. To chart out a workable training plan, you have to know yourself quite well, and for those of us who want a coach, we need to be able to form a strong relationship with that person.

I ultimately decided to provide training schedule examples because it's important for you to see all the run simple concepts come together in weeks and months, but I hope I've sufficiently warned you about them.

Sample Advanced Marathon Plan (16 Weeks)

Week	Mon	Tues	Wed	Thurs	Fri	Sat	Sun
1	JR: 50 min	JR: 40 min	JR: 50 min HH	JR: 40 min	JR: 50 min S 2x 2 min (middle)	JR: 40 min	JR: 60 min
2	JR: 60 min	JR: 40 min	JR: 72 min PROG	REST: M 40 min	JR: 80 min	REST: NW	JR: 90 min LR
3	JR: 50 min	JR: 72 min PROG	JR: 60 min	RACE: TR 3 x 1600m (6:00 recovery)	REST: NW	JR: 60 min	RACE: TU (5K) GP: W
4	REST: NW	RACE: TR 4 x 1600m (6:00 recovery)	REST: NW	RACE: TMP 30 min	JR: 70 min HH	JR: 60 min	JR: 90 min LR
5	REST: NW	RACE: TTG (9 holes)	JR: 50 min	RACE: TMP 40 min	JR: 60 min	JR: 90 min LR	REST: G 50 min
6	JR: 70 min	RACE: TR 5 x 1600m (6:00 recovery)	REST: NW	RACE: GP: W 5 miles	JR: 60 min HH	JR: 100 min LR	REST: NW
7	JR: 72 min PROG	RACE: TR 6 x 1600m (6:00 recovery)	REST: M 50 min	RACE: TMP 45 min EH	JR: 70 min	JR 110 min LR S 4 x3min (middle)	REST: G 50 min
8	JR: 70 min	RACE: TR 7 x 1600m (6:00 recovery)	REST: M 45 min	RACE: TTG (11 holes)	JR: 60 min	JR: 90 min LR	REST: NW
9	JR: 60 min	RACE: TR 3 x 3200m (11:00 recovery)	REST: M 50 min	RACE: GP: NW 7 mi EH	JR: 60 min	REST: G 50 min	JR: 110 min LR S 4 x 3min (last 30 min)
10	JR: 60 min	RACE: TR 4 x 3200m (10:00 recovery)	REST: NW	RACE: TTG (12 holes)	REST: NW	JR: LR 130 min	JR: 60 min
11	JR: 70 min	REST: NW	JR: 80 min	RACE: GP: W 9 mi EH	REST: NW	JR: 80 min	JR: LR 140 min
12	REST: G 45 min	RACE: TR 5 x 3200 (<10:00 recovery)	REST: NW	RACE: GP: W 11 mi	REST: NW	JR: LR 160 min	REST: M 50 min
13	JR: 80 min	RACE: TMP 40 min	REST: NW	RACE: TTG (12 holes)	REST: M 40 min	JR: 80 min	RACE: GP: W TU (half marathon)
14	REST: NW	RACE: TTG (8 holes)	REST: NW	RACE: GP: NW 15 mi	REST: M 40 min	REST: NW	JR: 180 min LR
15	REST: M 50 min	REST: M 45 min	RACE: GP: W 2 x 2 mi (with 2:00 recovery)	REST: NW	REST: NW	JR: 90 min LR	REST: NW
16	REST: NW	JR: 60 min S 3 x 2:00 (middle)	REST: NW	REST: M 40 min	REST: M 30 min	REST: M 20 min	Marathon

Training Schedule Legend

DO	Day Off	NW	No Watch
EH	End Hills	PROG	Progression Run
G	Green Run	S	Surges (when in the run to complete them)
GP: NW	Goal-Pace No watch	TMP	Tempo Run
GP: W	Goal-Pace With watch	TR	Track Repeats (recovery time between reps)
HH	Hidden Hills	TTG	Tee-to-Green (# holes)
JR	Just Run	TU	Tune-Up Race
LR	Long Run	WK	Walk
M	Mind Run		

Sample Intermediate Marathon Plan (16 Weeks)

Week	Mon	Tues	Wed	Thurs	Fri	Sat	Sun
1	REST: WK 40 min	JR: 30 min	JR: 40 min HH	JR: 40 min	JR: 40 min S 2 x 2 min (middle of run)	JR: 30 min	REST: WK 30 min
2	JR: 50 min	JR: 40 min	JR: 60 min PROG	REST: M 30 min	JR: 80 min	REST: NW	JR: 80 min
3	JR: 50 min	JR: 40 min	JR: 50 min	RACE: TR 3 x 1600m (7:00 recovery)	REST: M 30 min	JR: 50 min	RACE: TU (5K) GP: W
4	REST: NW	RACE: TR 4 x 1600m (7:00 recovery)	REST: NW	RACE: TMP 30 min	JR: 50 min HH	JR: 70 min	JR: 72 min PROG
5	REST: NW	RACE: TTG (5 holes)	JR: 40 min	RACE: GP: W 5 miles	JR: 50 min	JR: 90 min LR	REST: G 45 min
6	JR: 60 min	RACE: TR 4 x 1600m (7:00 recovery)	REST: NW	RACE: TMP 30 min EH	JR: 60 min HH	JR: 90 min LR	REST: NW
7	JR: 60 min PROG	RACE: TR 4 x 1600m (<7:00 recovery)	REST: M 45 min	RACE: GP: W 6 miles EH	JR: 60 min	JR: 90 min LR S 4 x 3 min (middle)	REST: G 50 min
8	JR: 60 min	RACE: TR 5 x 1600m (<7:00 recovery)	REST: M 45 min	RACE: TTG (9 holes)	JR: 70 min	JR: 100 min LR	REST: NW
9	JR: 60 min	RACE: TR 2 x 3200m (14:00 recovery)	REST: M 50 min	RACE: TMP 40 min EH	REST: G 50 min	JR: 70 min	JR: 110 min LR S 4 x 3 min (last 30 min)
10	JR: 60 min	RACE: TR 3 x 3200m (14:00 recovery)	REST: NW	RACE: TTG (9 holes)	REST: NW	JR: 130 min LR	JR: 60 min
11	JR: 70 min	REST: NW	JR: 60 min	RACE: GP: W 8 mi EH	REST: NW	JR: 70 min	JR: 120 min LR
12	REST: G 45 min	RACE: TR 4 x 3200 (<14:00 recovery)	REST: NW	RACE: TMP 45 min EH	REST: NW	JR: 150 min LR	REST: M 35 min
13	JR: 60 min	RACE: TMP 40 min	REST: M 40 min	RACE: TTG (9 holes)	REST: NW	JR: 80 min	RACE: GP: W TU (half marathon)
14	REST: NW	RACE: TTG (5 holes)	REST: NW	RACE: GP: NW 14 mi	REST: NW	REST: NW	JR: 180 min LR
15	REST: M 45 min	REST: M 40 min	REST: G 35 min	RACE: GP: W 2 x 2 mi (with 2:00 recovery)	REST: NW	JR: 90 min LR	REST: NW
16	REST: NW	JR: 60 min S 3 x 2:00 (middle)	REST: NW	REST: M 30 min	REST: M 25 min	REST: DO	Marathon

Run Simple

Sample Beginner Marathon Plan (16 Weeks)

Week	Mon	Tues	Wed	Thurs	Fri	Sat	Sun
1	REST: WK 30 min	REST: WK 30 min	REST: WK 30 min	JR: 30 min	JR: 35 min	REST: WK 30 min	REST: DO
2	JR: 40 min	REST: WK 35 min	JR: 39 min PROG	REST: WK 45 min	JR: 45 min	REST: NW	REST: DO
3	JR: 45 min	JR: 35 min	JR: 45 min	RACE: TR 2 x 1600m (9:00 recovery)	REST: M 30 min	JR: 70 min	RACE: TU (5K) GP: W
4	REST: NW	RACE: TR 3 x 1600m (9:00 recovery)	REST: NW	RACE: TMP 30 min	JR: 40 min HH	JR: 60 min PROG	REST: DO
5	REST: NW	RACE: TTG (3 holes)	JR: 40 min	RACE: GP: W 3 miles	JR: 40 min	JR: 72 min PROG	REST: NW
6	JR: 50 min	RACE: TR 4 x 1600m (9:00 recovery)	REST: NW	RACE: TMP 30 min EH	JR: 50 min HH	JR: 85 min	REST: DO
7	JR: 60 min PROG	RACE: TR 4 x 1600m (<9:00 recovery)	REST: M 40 min	RACE: GP: W 5 miles EH	JR: 60 min	JR 90 min LR S 4 x 2 min (middle)	REST: G 40 min
8	JR: 60 min	RACE: TR 5 x 1600m (<9:00 recovery)	REST: NW	RACE: TTG (5 holes)	JR: 60 min	JR: 100 min LR	REST: DO
9	JR: 50 min	RACE: TR 2 x 3200m (18:00 recovery)	REST: M 40 min	RACE: TMP 40 min	REST: G 50 min	JR: 70 min	JR: 110 min LR S 4 x 2 min (last 30 min)
10	JR: 50 min	RACE: TR 3 x 3200m (17:00 recovery)	REST: NW	RACE: TTG (7 holes)	REST: NW	JR: 130 min LR	REST: DO
11	JR: 60 min	REST: NW	JR: 50 min	RACE: GP: W 7 mi EH	REST: NW	JR: 60 min	JR: 140 min LR
12	REST: NW	RACE: TR 4 x 3200 (<17:00 recovery)	REST: NW	RACE: TMP 35 min EH	REST: DO	JR: 160 min LR	REST: DO
13	JR: 60 min	REST: NW	REST: M 40 min	RACE: TTG (9 holes)	REST: NW	REST: DO	RACE: GP: W (for 9 miles) TU (half marathon)
14	REST: NW	RACE: TTG (3 holes)	REST: NW	RACE: GP: NW 11 mi	REST: NW	REST: DO	JR: 180 min LR
15	REST: DO	REST: M 40 min	REST: G 35 min	RACE: GP: W 2 x 2 mi (2:00 recovery)	REST: NW	JR: 50 min	REST: DO
16	REST: NW	JR: 45 min S 3 x 1 min	REST: NW	REST: M 30 min	REST: M 20 min	REST: DO	Marathon

Sample Advanced Half Marathon Plan (12 Weeks)

Week	Mon	Tues	Wed	Thurs	Fri	Sat	Sun
1	JR: 40 min	JR: 35 min	JR: 45 min HH	JR: 35 min	JR: 50 min S 2 x 2 min (anytime during run)	JR: 40 min	REST: M 30 min
2	JR: 50 min	JR: 30 min	JR: 60 min PROG	REST: M 40 min	JR: 50 min	REST: NW	JR: 50 min
3	JR: 40 min	JR: 30 min	JR: 60 min	RACE: TR 3 x 800m (3:00 recovery)	REST: M 30 min	JR: 30 min	RACE: TU (5K) GP: W
4	REST: NW	RACE: TR 4 x 800m (2:30 recovery)	REST: NW	RACE: TMP 25 min	JR: 40 min HH	JR: 50 min	JR: 72 min PROG
5	REST: NW	RACE: TTG (4 holes)	JR: 50 min	RACE: GP: W 4 miles	JR: 50 min	JR: 60 min	REST: G 45 min
6	JR: 50 min	RACE: TR 5 x 800m (2:30 recovery)	REST: NW	RACE: TMP 30 min EH	JR: 50 min HH	JR: 90 min LR	REST: NW
7	JR: 60 min PROG	RACE: TR 6 x 800m (2:30 recovery)	REST: M 50 min	RACE: GP: NW 7 miles EH	JR: 50 min	JR 100 min LR S 4 x 3 min (middle)	REST: G 40 min
8	JR: 70 min	RACE: TR 7 x 800m (2:30 recovery)	REST: M 40 min	RACE: TTG (5 holes)	JR: 60 min	JR: 90 min LR	REST: NW
9	JR: 60 min	RACE: TR 3 x 1600m (6:00 recovery)	REST: M 50 min	RACE: TMP 40 min EH	JR: 60 min	REST: G 40 min	RACE: TU (10K) GP: W
10	REST: NW	RACE: TR 5 x 1600m (6:00 recovery)	REST: M 50 min	RACE: GP: W 9 miles EH	REST: NW	JR: 100 min LR	REST: NW
11	REST: M 35 min	REST: M 35 min	REST: G 40 min	RACE: TMP 40 min EH	REST: NW	JR: 90 min LR	REST: NW
12	REST: NW	JR: 50 min S 3 x 2:00 (end of run)	REST: NW	REST: M 35 min	REST: M 25 min	REST: DO	Half Marathon

Run Simple

Sample Intermediate Half Marathon Plan (12 Weeks)

Week	Mon	Tues	Wed	Thurs	Fri	Sat	Sun
1	REST: WK 40 min	JR: 35 min	JR: 40 min HH	JR: 35 min	JR: 50 min S 2 x 2 min (anytime during run)	JR: 40 min	REST: DO
2	JR: 40 min	JR: 30 min	JR: 60 min PROG	REST: M 40 min	JR: 50 min	REST: NW	JR: 50 min
3	JR: 40 min	JR: 30 min	JR: 60 min	RACE: TR 3 x 800m (4:00 recovery)	REST: M 30 min	REST: NW	RACE: TU (5K) GP: W
4	REST: NW	RACE: TR 4 x 800m (3:30 recovery)	REST: NW	RACE: TMP 20 min	JR: 40 min HH	JR: 30 min	JR: 72 min PROG
5	REST: NW	RACE: TTG (3 holes)	JR: 50 min	RACE: GP: W 4 miles	REST: NW	JR: 50 min	REST: G 35 min
6	JR: 50 min	RACE: TR 3 x 800m (3:30 recovery)	REST: NW	RACE: TMP 25 min EH	REST: NW	JR: 90 min LR	REST: NW
7	JR: 60 min PROG	RACE: TR 4 x 800m (3:30 recovery)	REST: M 35 min	RACE: GP: NW 6 miles EH	JR: 40 min	JR 100 min LR S 4 x 2 min (middle)	REST: G 40 min
8	JR: 60 min	RACE: TR 5 x 800m (3:30 recovery)	REST: M 40 min	RACE: TTG (4 holes)	JR: 50 min	JR: 90 min LR	REST: NW
9	JR: 60 min	RACE: TR 2 x 1600m (7:00 recovery)	REST: M 45 min	RACE: TMP 35 min EH	JR: 60 min	REST: G 35 min	RACE: TU (10K) GP: W
10	REST: NW	RACE: TR 3 x 1600m (7:00 recovery)	REST: M 40 min	RACE: TMP 45 min EH	REST: NW	JR: 100 min LR	REST: NW
11	REST: M 45 min	REST: M 40 min	REST: G 40 min	RACE: GP: W 8 miles	REST: NW	JR: 90 min LR	REST: NW
12	REST: NW	JR: 50 min S 3 x 2:00 (end of run)	REST: NW	REST: M 30 min	REST: M 20 min	REST: DO	Half Marathon

Sample Beginner Half Marathon Plan (12 Weeks)

Week	Mon	Tues	Wed	Thurs	Fri	Sat	Sun
1	REST: WK 30 min	REST: WK 30 min	JR: 30 min HH	REST: WK 30 min	JR: 35 min S 2 x 1:30 (anytime during run)	JR: 40 min	REST: DO
2	REST: WK 35 min	JR: 30 min	JR: 39 min PROG	REST: M 30 min	JR: 40 min	REST: NW	REST: DO
3	JR: 40 min	JR: 30 min	JR: 40 min HH	RACE: TR 2 x 800m (5:00 recovery)	REST: M 30 min	REST: NW	RACE: TU (5K) GP: W
4	REST: NW	RACE: TR 4 x 800m (3:30 recovery)	REST: NW	RACE: TMP 20 min	JR: 40 min HH	JR: 30 min	REST: DO
5	REST: NW	RACE: TTG (3 holes)	REST: NW	RACE: GP: NW 3 miles	REST: NW	JR: 50 min	REST: G 35 min
6	JR: 50 min	RACE: TR 3 x 800m (5:00 recovery)	REST: NW	RACE: TMP 25 min EH	REST: NW	JR: 60 min	REST: DO
7	JR: 54 min PROG	RACE: TR 4 x 800m (4:30 recovery)	REST: NW	RACE: GP: W 5 miles EH	JR: 40 min	JR 70 min S 4 x 2 min (middle)	REST: DO
8	JR: 50 min	RACE: TR 5 x 800m (4:30 recovery)	REST: M 30 min	RACE: TTG (4 holes)	JR: 50 min	JR: 90 min LR	REST: DO
9	JR: 50 min	RACE: TR 2 x 1600m (9:00 recovery)	REST: M 40 min	RACE: TMP 35 min EH	JR: 60 min	REST: DO	RACE: TU (10K) GP: W
10	REST: NW	RACE: TR 3 x 1600m (9:00 recovery)	REST: M 30 min	RACE: GP: NW 7 miles	REST: NW	JR: 100 min LR	REST: DO
11	REST: M 45 min	REST: M 40 min	REST: G 35 min	RACE: TMP 40 min EH	REST: NW	JR: 50 min	REST: DO
12	REST: NW	JR: 50 min S 3 x1:00 (end of run)	REST: NW	REST: M 25 min	REST: M 20 min	REST: DO	Half Marathon

Sample Advanced 5K/10K Plan (8 Weeks)

Week	Mon	Tues	Wed	Thurs	Fri	Sat	Sun
1	JR: 40 min	JR: 30 min	JR: 40 min HH	JR: 30 min	JR: 50 min S 2 x 1:00 (anytime during run)	JR: 40 min	JR: 60 min PROG
2	JR: 50 min	JR: 40 min	JR: 60 min PROG	JR: 50 min HH	JR: 40 min	JR: 50 min	REST: NW
3	JR: 50 min	JR: 40 min	JR: 40 min HH	RACE: TR 5 x 400m (1:00 recovery)	REST: M 40 min	JR: 50 min	JR: 70 min
4	REST: NW	RACE: TR 6 x 400m (1:00 recovery)	REST: NW	RACE: TMP 30 min	JR: 60 min HH	JR: 40 min	JR: 81 min PROG
5	REST: NW	RACE: TTG (6 holes)	JR: 40 min	RACE: TMP 35 min EH	JR: 30 min	JR: 90 min I.R	REST: G 25 min
6	JR: 50 min	RACE: TR 8 x 400m (1:00 recovery)	REST: NW	RACE: TR 10 x 400m (1:00 recovery)	REST: NW	JR: 70 min	REST: M 35 min
7	JR: 60 min PROG	RACE: TR 5 x 800m (2:00 recovery)	REST: M 30 min	RACE: TMP 40 min EH	JR: 40 min	JR 60 min S 6 x 1 min (middle)	REST: DO
8	REST: NW	JR: 30 min S 3 x 1:00 (end of run)	REST: NW	REST: M 30 min	REST: M 20 min	REST: DO	5K/10K

Sample Intermediate 5K/10K Plan (8 Weeks)

Week	Mon	Tues	Wed	Thurs	Fri	Sat	Sun
1	REST: WK 30 min	JR: 20 min	JR: 30 min HH	JR: 20 min	JR: 35 min S 2 x 1:00 (anytime during run)	JR: 40 min	JR: 30 min
2	JR: 40 min	JR: 35 min	JR: 42 min PROG	JR: 30 min HH	JR: 30 min	REST: NW	REST: DO
3	JR: 40 min	JR: 30 min	JR: 35 min	RACE: TR 4 x 400m (1:30 recovery)	REST: M 30 min	JR: 30 min	JR: 60 min
4	REST: NW	RACE: TR 4 x 400m (1:30 recovery)	REST: NW	RACE: TMP 25 min	JR: 30 min HH	JR: 20 min	REST: DO
5	REST: NW	RACE: TTG (4 holes)	JR: 40 min	RACE: TMP 30 min EH	JR: 30 min	JR: 50 min	REST: G 25 min
6	JR: 40 min	RACE: TR 4 x 400m (1:30 recovery)	REST: NW	RACE: TR 6 x 400m (1:30 recovery)	REST: NW	JR: 50 min	REST: DO
7	JR: 42 min PROG	RACE: TR 3 x 800m (3:00 recovery)	REST: M 20 min	RACE: TMP 35 min EH	JR: 40 min	JR 60 min S 4 x 1 min (middle)	REST: DO
8	REST: NW	JR: 30 min S 3 x 1:00 (end of run)	REST: NW	REST: M 25 min	REST: M 20 min	REST: DO	5K/10K

Sample Beginner 5K/10K Plan (8 Weeks)

Week	Mon	Tues	Wed	Thurs	Fri	Sat	Sun
1	REST: WK 20 min	REST: WK 20 min	JR: 25 min HH	REST: DO	JR: 35 min S 2 x 1:00 (anytime during run)	JR: 30 min	REST: DO
2	REST: WK 20 min	JR: 35 min	JR:36 min PROG	REST: DO	JR: 30 min	REST: NW	REST: DO
3	REST: WK 20 min	JR: 30 min	JR: 35 min	RACE: TR 3 x 400m (2:00 recovery)	REST: NW	JR: 30 min	REST: DO
4	REST: NW	RACE: TR 3 x 400m (2:00 recovery)	REST: NW	REST: DO	JR: 30 min HH	JR: 20 min	REST: DO
5	REST: NW	RACE: TTG (3 holes)	JR: 30 min	RACE: TMP 20 min EH	JR: 30 min	JR: 45 min PROG	REST: G 25 min
6	JR: 50 min	RACE: TR 4 x 400m (2:00 recovery)	REST: NW	Rest: Day Off	JR: 40 min HH	JR: 30 min	REST: DO
7	JR: 36 min PROG	RACE: TR 3 x 800m (4:00 recovery)	REST: NW	RACE: TMP 20 min EH	JR: 40 min	JR 60 min S 4 x 1 min (middle)	REST: DO
8	REST: NW	JR: 30 min S 3 x 30 sec (end of run)	REST: NW	REST: M 25 min	REST: M 20 min	REST: DO	5K/10K

How to Create Your Own Schedule

At this point you should create your own customized plan. You know your body and schedule better than I do. The following graphical representation of the run simple training elements can help you chart out your own schedule:

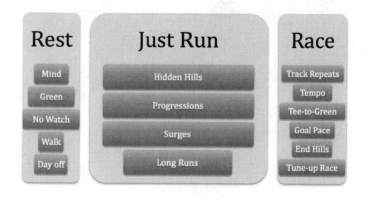

These specific phases can be further summarized as follows:

Rest

Type	Goal	Pace	Specific Stimulus
Mind	Relaxation and recovery	Slow	Spend the entire run only thinking positive thoughts about life and your upcoming race
Green	Taking the focus off yourself	Slow	Picking up roadside trash or doing other selfless activities
No Watch	Not stressing about time and pace	Slow	No stimulus. Total relaxation
Walk	Weight loss and building leg strength in addition to giving the legs a break from running	Slow (doesn't have to be race walking)	Just getting out and moving the legs. Enjoy the scenery.
Day off	Don't run or walk	N/A	A day off is a day off. Don't overachieve. Do nothing.

Just Run

Type	Goal	Pace	Specific Stimulus
Hidden Hills	Finding new routes with hills you didn't know about.	Moderate until you reach the surprise hill.	Work the legs, ankles, and lungs when you encounter a hill. Simulate race-day chaos and unplanned moves made by opponents.
Surges	Sudden and rapid increases of pace in the middle of your run.	All out. As fast as you can tolerate for the designated time period.	More race-day simulation of chaos; simulating a move. Preparing the body to react to the suddenness that can occur when goal pace is missed on race day.
Long Run	Getting as much time on your feet as possible.	Of no concern.	Building leg strength, increasing efficiency, and adapting to the stresses of sustained running > 90 minutes.
Progression	Gradual increase of pace throughout the run.	Break the workout into thirds; run the first third slow, the second third medium, and last third all out.	Safe way to incorporate faster-paced running by using the run to warm up the body.

Race

Type	Goal	Pace	Specific Stimulus
Tempo Runs	Run at a quick pace for a sustained period of time.	10K race pace	The entire run should be challenging. You should be breathing and working hard.
Tee-to-Green	Simulate the chaotic nature of a race while having some fun	As fast as possible between "holes"	Learning how to cope with the "randomness" of a race in terms of pace and distance.
End Hills	Plan your route on this day to finish up a hill.	All out, attack the hill!	Working your ankles, lungs, and legs. It's also a challenge to encounter additional resistance at the end of an already-difficult workout.
Goal Pace	Complete the required time/distance at your goal race pace. Some days you wear a watch and consult it at every mile split. Some days you don't look at it until the end.	The exact pace you expect to run come race day	Your most important workout. You are preparing the mind and body for the rigors required to achieve your goal. Use these workouts later in your schedule to understand if your goals are realistic.
Tune-up Race	Compete in a local race	Depends, but no slower than your goal race pace	The ultimate aim is to practice racing and experiment with running at or faster than your goal race pace.

And finally, some pointers on how to build out your customized schedule:

Practice Gradualism

When it's time to chart out your schedule, make everything at the beginning of the plan less in terms of duration and repeats. So, for your track repeats, begin them with three or four and then increase in number by one or two repeats every week. Same goes for your long runs: don't throw in a 90-minute run when the longest you've run before was only 40 minutes. Build up everything slowly. If you are starting the plan with a decent aerobic base, then it's OK to jump into your Race runs, but if you've taken a long break from running, build up your training with a lot of Rest and easy Just Run workouts.

Give Yourself Equal Time or Less for Your Track Repeats

You get no recovery time between miles in your race, so try to give yourself as little opportunity to rest when you are on the track doing your faster-than-goal-pace repeats. Ratchet back the recovery time as much as possible. Obviously, it depends on the length of the repeat, but an example would be giving yourself 5 minutes of recovery after conducting 7-minute, 1,600-meter repeats.

Make Your Track Repeats Longer If Your Goal Race Is Longer

If you are training for 5K-10Ks, work on quarters (one lap) and 800s (two laps). If you're going for a half-marathon goal, increase the distance of your repeats to a mile. Marathoners should also be completing mile repeats at first, but try to move up to two-mile repeats later in the schedule. This guidance isn't fixed in stone. Arguments can be made for marathoners doing quarters every once in a while, so experiement and mix it up if you are getting bored doing the same type of repeat. You can also incorporate "ladders" into your routine. These are a mixture of repeats at various distances within the same session. They usually start with shorter reps gradually building in distance until a maximum is achieved, then they decline in distance back to the starting point. A sample ladder routine could be: 1 x 400m, 1 x 800m, 1 x 1200m, 1 x 1600m, 1 x 1200m, 1 x 800m, 1 x 400m. Ladders are nice because they mix up pace and distance. They also give you a goal to strive for. In the previous example, that goal would be making it to the 1600m repeat, knowing that every repeat after that point will be shorter in distance. That can be encouraging in a hard session, compared to someome stuck doing 4 x 1600m, with the understanding that each distance run is exactly the same.

Try to Schedule Rest Days after Your Race Days

You have to give yourself time to recover. Don't try to put in two Race days in a row. If you want to Just Run the day after a workout, make it something short and relatively easy. Your body needs and deserves the rest.

Build Comfort Running at Your Goal Pace

Slowly and gradually sprinkle in your goal-pace-specific Race workouts. Understand that Goal Pace may be difficult at first, so take that into account in the beginning of your plan. For marathoners and half marathoners, try to get to the point where you can successfully run over half the total goal-race time at your goal pace in training. Even better if you can cover three-quarters of the time–that should be your ultimate aim. When you begin to fill in your customized training schedule, try to start with these all-important workouts. And then when you think you have your schedule complete, after you've tweaked various workouts, revisit the goal-pace aspect of it one more time. Ask yourself these questions:

How much goal-pace work am I doing in the total schedule?

How much goal-pace work am I doing each week?

What are the differences in goal-pace duration (mileage or time) from one workout to the next and from week to week?

What is the maximum goal-pace workout I'm completing in the schedule, and how much time am I giving myself before I start my taper?

Use the Goals of the Specific Workouts to Develop Areas You Think Need Work

Before you chart out your schedule, do some serious introspection. As a racer, what are you good at? What needs work? What doesn't need work? If, for example, you always go out too fast at the beginning and run out of gas, so that you get passed by your competitors at the end, commit to focusing on controlling your effort and improving your pace discipline. Progression runs are great for this; so are Goal-Pace runs. On the other side of the spectrum, you may feel like you are heading into your races or workouts always burned out. You doubt your abilities and even question why it is you are running in the first place. Sounds like it's time for a couple of Rest days.

Make Good Use of Your Just Run Days

Since these are the foundational elements of your schedule, make them count. This doesn't mean you run them all hard; it means you use them to work on specific things. If you know your upcoming 5K is going to be on a hilly course, for example, throw several Hidden Hills routines into your schedule before the race.

Don't Forget to Include a Taper

Every schedule should allow you to slowly build up your mileage as well as your hard-effort sessions (in terms of number of repetitions, length of long run, and length of repetitions). However, you need to give your body time to recover from all this work. Optimally, a marathon schedule tapers two weeks beforehand and a half marathon one week beforehand; for a 5K/10K, give yourself at least three to four days of taper.

When You Taper, Do It Properly

When you are building taper into your schedule, ensure

the majority of your days are Rest runs. Since you are gearing up for your big race, make them Mind runs and practice positive visualization constantly as you are tapering. Imagine feeling good come race day, and tell yourself you are going to run your goal. Every few days of your taper, it's good to incorporate some Goal Pace workouts to get the body used to the pace it will run on race day. But no matter what, err on the side of caution during your taper. You don't want to show up on race day with tired legs. You have worked hard going into the taper and deserve to take it easy.

Build in Rest Weeks

Not only do you need to plan for proper rest within your week, but you also need to look at incorporating rest as the goal of the week itself. A good rule of thumb is to back off in terms of effort and duration once every three weeks. Your Rest week should obviously have more Rest days than a usual training week. And it's OK to have one Race workout, but make it shorter in duration, volume, and distance than your other Race workouts.

Focus on What Needs Work

If you aren't new to running and this isn't your first training schedule, then you should take a moment to think about yourself as a runner before you chart it out. Ask yourself what areas you believe you need to develop. Where were you challenged in your last goal race? If the final 10K of the marathon was abysmal, put in a lot of longer, faster runs in your training schedule. Work to develop comfort at your goal pace; make your tempo runs longer and try to run as many goal-pace miles in a row as you can stomach. If you got passed on a long hill, add a lot of End Hills and Hidden Hills workouts into your schedule. If you are starting out a new schedule with a decent cardiovascular base and your legs are already strong, then ramp up the work on your schedule quicker. Make the progression in terms of volume, distance, and pace steeper than if you were beginning the schedule as someone who's taken a long break from running.

A Final Word for Beginning Runners

If you are completely new to running, you may be getting overwhelmed at this point. You might not even know where to begin as you create your first customized schedule. Remember, the formula doesn't make the runner. A schedule is a rough guide. Don't get consumed by it. Start out using the Beginner schedule in this book and then apply common sense as you become wiser about your limitations and abilities. Be realistic with your goals and be patient. As your body begins to adapt to running, you will experience physical and mental setbacks. To best prepare for these, don't waste too much time laying out a long, detailed schedule. Just write out the first two to three weeks and include a lot of Rest runs and easy Just Run workouts. Your first few training weeks may be focused on losing weight and building up muscular strength and endurance (versus running a certain time goal in a race). If that's the case, give yourself a checkpoint where you will switch goals and create a fresh schedule.

four

Quit the Gym

ALMOST EVERY TOWN—LARGE OR SMALL—HAS A GYM, and that gym has a staff of membership-oriented sales folks who have one mission: seduce as many people as possible into signing up with them. These folks are no different than car salesmen. They thrive on quotas. The more paying customers they can get into the door, the better. You may seem to matter to them, but you're just a number. Whatever you tell them about yourself they will most likely twist into a convincing-sounding argument for why you should hand over your credit card and sign a contract. Money matters. You're a means to an end. Once they glean the information from you that you're a runner, they will typically show you all the expensive cardio machines as part of their sales pitch.

"Where will you run when it rains?" they will ask.

"What happens if you get injured?"

"We have plenty of low-impact machines for you!"

Their expensive cardio rooms will undoubtedly be filled with blaring television sets. Stuffed magazine racks will be an arm's reach away from the treadmills.

Gyms are all about eye-catching distraction. Watch television while you run. Read while you run. Gaze at others while you run. Do anything but be at peace with yourself while you run. This place isn't where you run simple; there is no soothing silence here. This place is a giant, circus-like room designed for the modern person with no attention span–the person who needs to be constantly entertained and overstimulated.

That's not you, is it?

The salespeople will then walk you past rooms filled with muscled people squatting and heaving next to various daunting free weights and other complicated resistance equipment. Most gym sales pitches end with signing perks, like a free month of membership, or three free spinning classes if you sign the contract today. Even with those perks, gym membership packages typically run anywhere from $100 a month to as much as $300.

You're a runner. Do you really need to go to one of these places?

Are they worth paying up to $3,600 a year to visit?

Practically everything you need to successfully cross-train for running can be found either on your body or in your home. And the only out-of-pocket investment entails shelling out about $10.

Before I get into some simple exercises, it's important to explain why you need to do them. First, a runner with lean, strong muscles (not large, bulky muscles) is usually a faster runner. And second, a runner who's been consistently cross-training these muscles is a runner with a greater potential of staying injury-free.

The running muscles you need to develop that we'll talk about in this chapter can be broken down into two groups: core and supplemental.

Core Muscles

Just what are your core muscles, and why is it important as a runner to keep them strong?

In order to run well, your body depends on these stabilizing muscles to keep it upright and balanced. Running is an incredibly complex movement for us bipeds, and the body has to work constantly to prevent it from falling over. Theoretically, the stronger these important muscles are, the less prone you are to being injured, and a well-developed core can even aid in running faster and more efficiently.

It's not that important to know all the muscles that make up your core. After all, you're a runner, not an exercise physiologist. It is important, however, to know that, contrary to conventional wisdom, your core muscles are not just your abdominals. They include numerous muscles and muscle groups in your hips and pelvic floor. There are even core muscles buried under other muscles.

Supplemental Muscles

Along with the all-important core group, a runner should also pay attention to strengthening supplemental muscles, such as those in the arms and chest.

Why?

Consider this: the next time you need something to ponder during your run, count how many times you swing your arms. Every time you swing your arms, your biceps, triceps, chest, and back are hard at work pushing and pulling the arm forward and backward. Lean but strong arm and chest muscles make it easier for you to run. Neck and arm cramps won't form. Your stride will become more efficient, and you will have an easier time staying balanced.

Now Off to the Five-Dollar Store!

The most important item you will need to exercise at home is a stability ball, which is a giant round piece of plastic that you inflate. Stability balls–also called exercise balls or Swiss balls–are probably the best piece of exercise equipment out there. Typically they come in three sizes: 22 inches (55cm), 26 inches (65cm), and 30 inches (75cm). The right size for you depends on your height (22 inches if you're under 5 foot 5, 26 inches if you're between 5 foot

6 and 6 feet, and 30 inches if you're over 6 feet tall).

Near where I live, there's a chain of stores called Five Below, named for the fact that everything there costs under $5. These stores typically stock stability balls. If you don't have a Five Below in your area, plenty of other discount stores sell them. Five Below also happens to sell dumbbells, which is the second item you will need for these workouts.

If you aren't into buying new things made in China, you can most likely find these items at a garage sale or on Craigslist. Also, keep an eye out for gyms that are closing in your area. They usually have fire sales. Another option is to borrow them from a friend. There are plenty of people out there not using their fitness equipment.

The weight of the dumbbell you need depends on how strong you currently are. But a word of caution: you don't want to become muscle-bound. These are supplemental activities with the primary goals of warding off injury and getting you to run more efficiently. For the exercises that this book prescribes, err on the side of buying a lighter dumbbell. This is because you will be completing more repetitions with lighter weight instead of heavier weight and fewer repetitions. Lighter weights combined with increased repetitions tones the muscle as opposed to building it up. Muscle mass is heavy. As a distance runner, you don't want that extra weight. You want to be as svelte as possible.

To find the right dumbbell weight for you, start out with something you can comfortably lift but that causes you to experience fatigue after 15 to 20 repetitions of an exercise (for example, a bicep curl). Buy two dumbbells of that weight and then buy two more dumbbells of the next lighter weight.

What follows is a detailed description and depiction of the cross-training exercises you will be completing in the four-week schedule:

The Plank

What it is	Holding your body in position for a designated period of time. Theoretically, the longer you can hold that position, the better.
What it works	Abdominals, back, legs, and arms. This is pretty much the best possible all-around exercise. I love it. You don't need any equipment. You can "plank" pretty much anywhere.
What you need	Nothing other than a soft surface and a watch. Even if you don't have a watch, you can count out the seconds.
How to do it	Start on your hands and knees. Then extend your legs similar to a push up, but rest your weight on the balls of your toes and your forearms. Don't let yourself sag too much.
	An alternative to the regular Plank is called an "Around the World Plank". Start the same as you do for the regular Plank, but for 30-second intervals lift up either one hand or one leg (alternating between sides) at a 45-degree angle until you have raised each appendage once.

What it looks like

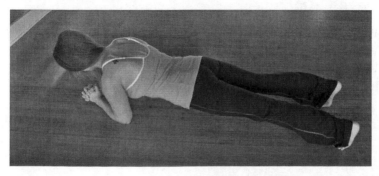

Side Plank

What it is   Another variation of the plank exercise
What it works   Abdominals, back, legs and arms
What you need   Nothing other than a soft surface
How to do it   Start the same as the plank, but rotate
                    your body so that your hips face the
                    wall instead of the floor. Reach up with
                    one hand at a 45-degree angle towards
                    the ceiling. Hold this for 30 seconds and
                    then switch sides.
What it looks like

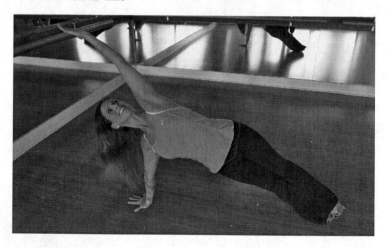

Devil Crunch

What it is   A challenging abdominal exercise
What it works   Abdominals
What you need   Soft surface to lie down on
How to do it   Lie flat on your back and put your
                    hands behind your head. Bring your
                    head up like a normal crunch, but at the
                    same time, bring your legs up as well

such that your knees touch your elbows. Hold this for five seconds then return to the starting position; however, do not let your legs touch the ground between repetitions.

Why is it called the Devil Crunch? When I was in the army, my brigade commander invented this exercise. Our unit was the 504th Parachute Infantry Regiment (nicknamed the "Devils in Baggy Pants"), hence the "devil" reference. But when you are doing them you may feel like the devil is standing on you.

What it looks like

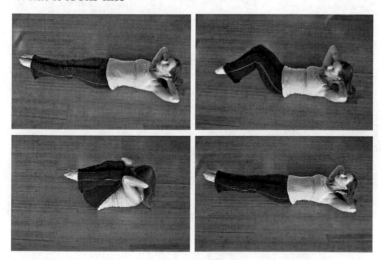

Bicycle Crunches

What it is	Besides the plank, one of the best abdominal workouts there is
What it works	Abdominals
What you need	A soft surface to lie down on
How to do it	Lie on your back. Raise your feet six inches off the ground. Put your hands behind your head. Touch one elbow to the opposite knee, return to starting position and then touch the other elbow to the opposite knee. Repeat. Don't let your feet touch the ground.

What it looks like

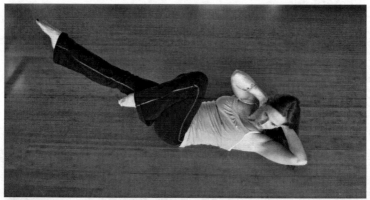

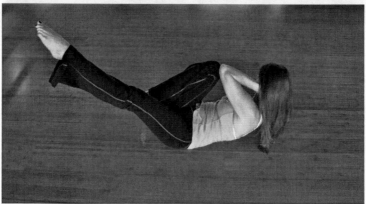

Flutter Kicks and Hello Dollies

What it is	Two abdominal workouts
What it works	Abdominals
What you need	A soft surface to lie down on
How to do it	For both Flutter Kicks and Hello Dollies lie on your back with your feet straight. Raise your feet six inches off the ground. For Flutter Kicks move your feet up and down while not touching the ground. For Hello Dollies, move your legs side to side. Never touch the ground in either instance. Try to keep your legs as straight as possible.

What it looks like (Flutter Kicks)

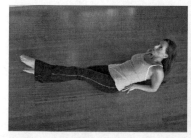 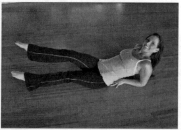

What it looks like (Hello Dollies)

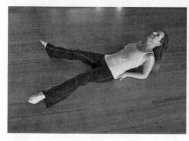 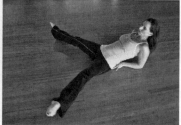

Twenty-Ones

What it is	A variation of the standard bicep curl that integrates repetition with a little fun.
What it works	Biceps and forearms
What you need	Two lighter dumbbells
How to do it	Stand with feet shoulder length apart. Perform 21 repetitions with each arm in the following manner—the first seven repetitions bring the dumbbell from rest position to a 90-degree angle. For the second of seven repetitions, bring the dumbbell from a 90-degree angle all the way up to your bicep. Your last seven repetitions are then the standard bicep curl (from the rest position all the way up).

What it looks like

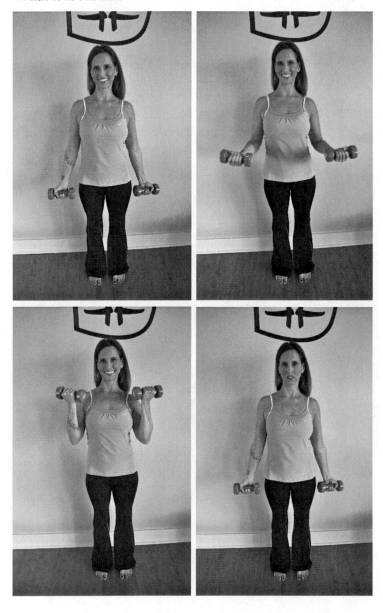

Hammer Curls

What it is   A variation of the standard bicep curl
What it works   Biceps and forearms
What you need   Stability ball and two lighter dumbbells
How to do it   Sit on the stability ball. Keeping your
                    back straight bring the dumbbells up as
                    if you were doing a curl, but don't hold
                    the dumbbell out across your palm like
                    a traditional bicep curl. Instead, grab it
                    as if you were holding a baton.

What it looks like

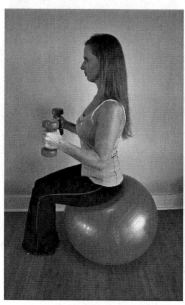 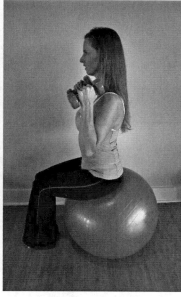

Seated Row

What it is   A simple back exercise

What it works   Back and shoulders

What you need   Stability ball and your two lighter-weight dumbbells

How to do it   Sit on the Stability ball. Bend forwards slightly while raising your arms close to your sides. Bend at the elbow with the elbow close to your ribs and then drop your arms to the starting position. Try to keep your elbows parallel with the ceiling.

What it looks like

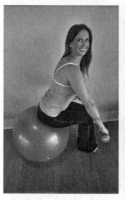 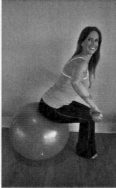 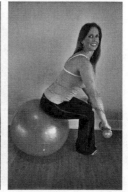

Triceps Extensions

What it is	A simple workout to isolate your triceps
What it works	Triceps
What you need	One heavy dumbbell
How to do it	Stand with your feet shoulder-length apart or alternatively you can sit on a stability ball. Taking one dumbbell in both hands, raise it above your head and slowly bring it down behind you. Don't let the dumbbell touch your back during the repetition.

What it looks like

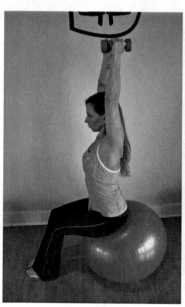 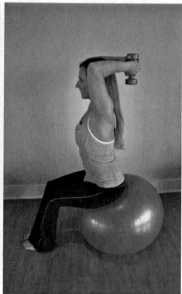

Seated Dips

What it is	A variation of the elevated dip
What it works	Chest, forearms, and triceps
What you need	Side of a bed or couch
How to do it	Put your back up against the object while placing your arms behind you. Rest your hands on the object with your fingers facing forward. Raise yourself up and then lower yourself down as far as possible without touching the floor with your buttocks. Push yourself back up for one repetition.

What it looks like

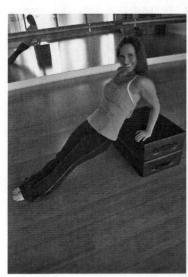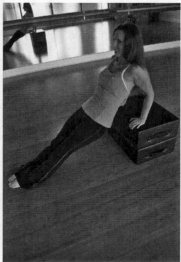

Balanced Push ups

What it is   A variation of the standard pushup

What it works   Chest and triceps. This exercise also can
                  work your core as you try to maintain
                  your balance.

What you need   A stability ball or the side of a bed or
                  couch

How to do it   Place your feet up on the stability ball
                  and walk out to the pushup position.
                  Complete normal pushups while staying
                  balanced. For variation and to work
                  different muscle groups, change the
                  width between your hands.

What it looks like

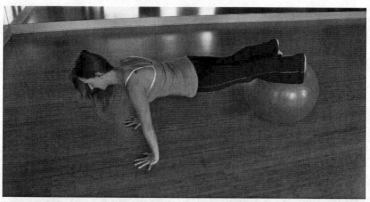

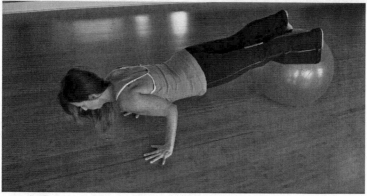

Bench Press on Ball

What it is	Bench press while laying on a stability ball
What it works	Chest and triceps
What you need	A stability ball and your heavier dumbbell
How to do it	Lie on your back using the stability ball to hold you up. Keep your knees bent and your feet flat on the floor. Using two dumbbells, palms facing towards the ceiling lower the dumbbells simultaneously until the dumbbells are even with your ears and then return them to the starting position for one repetition.

What it looks like

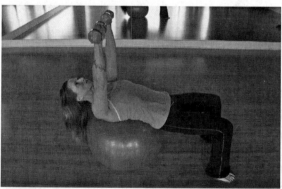

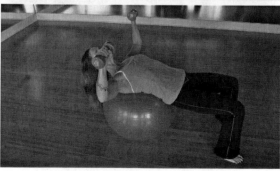

This Isn't a Race!

Take your time doing these exercises. Rushing through the routines isn't going to make you stronger. It might even cause an injury, so when you are making your way through the repetitions, count them out loud and keep telling yourself to slow down. Gently exhale as you complete each repetition. When you start to feel pain, you may be tempted to rush your way to completion.

Don't.

If you can't complete the prescribed number of repetitions in the schedule, that's OK. Do as many as you can and don't beat yourself up about it. Take a brief rest and then resume until you finish. The more you do these things, the easier it will get.

Be patient.

Alternative Exercises

So what if you don't have a stability ball or a pair of dumbbells? Plenty of objects in your house (or hotel room) work fine as substitutes. The side of a bed or a sofa can serve as alternative equipment when you don't have a stability ball. You can prop your feet up on these items to achieve elevation, so a rather routine set of pushups could be made more interesting by elevating every other set. You can also do seated dips using the side of a bed.

If you don't have dumbbells handy, be creative. Canned goods (for example, heavy soups, or vegetables like beans) can act as a substitute. And if you have nothing, there's always your own weight. You can do the plank exercise explained in this chapter, and do pushups/dips pretty much anywhere.

Make Good Use of Your Cubicle

Bring your stability ball and dumbbells to work with you. Every hour or so, sit on your stability ball for 10 to 15 minutes. It's a great way to work your core muscles. When the mood strikes you, pull out your dumbbells and do a few

exercises found in this book. Just having these items in your cubicle or office will make your work more interesting.

Stay Active While Traveling

If you are ever traveling on business and staying in a hotel, there is no excuse not to work out. Business travelers are usually stuck in the same chain-type hotel near an airport with *USA Today* delivered to their doors every morning. After the meetings and mandatory socializing is complete, the tired travelers all go to the same chain restaurants and then walk back to their hotel rooms, where most of them watch TV before going to bed.

Don't be like them.

Understandably, business travel is tiring, but you should find the energy to work out—every day. The next time you travel on business, go exploring. Limitless new running routes are out there waiting for you. And if you don't have your trusty stability ball and dumbbells with you, there's no shame in visiting the hotel gym and doing your cross-training there. Most hotel gyms have these items. If going to the hotel gym is not for you, then incorporate some simple exercises in your hotel room, like balanced pushups, plank, and bedside dips.

When Is the Best Time to Work Out?

There is only so much time in the day to devote to physical fitness. Therefore, other than doing exercises like planking and pushups on the fly, try to integrate your running and cross-training. The best time to cross-train is after you run. Your body is warmed up. Endorphins are flowing in your veins. You may be tired, but you should be happy that you've done something worthwhile in the day. And logistically speaking, you're already sweaty and smelly. Spending 10 more minutes working your upper body and core won't make things any worse on that front.

After taking a drink and walking a bit, get down to business and complete your required cross-training exercises.

Be sure not to cross-train before a key "Race" workout, like a track repeat session or a tempo run—something that requires every ounce of your energy. Remember that above all else, running is the top priority. Do the running first and the cross-training later.

Thirty Days of Cross-Training Explained

Just like the running schedules, what follows is a suggested plan that integrates the exercises and concepts you've just learned. Since each person picking up this book is at a different stage of upper and lower body fitness, it's nearly impossible to suggest the exact number of repetitions to complete or the precise weight of dumbbells for you to use. Therefore, take this schedule as an example of how to put everything together.

The schedule should motivate you to do *something* after your arduous run. As currently written, the 30-day schedule is probably best suited for someone not prone to working out frequently, since it starts relatively easy.

Once a week, on Saturdays, you will be competing against yourself for personal records. Like chasing after a goal with your running, go for records with cross-training. So let's see how long you can plank. Compare your time on week one to week four. Write down how many pushups you can complete without going to your knees for rest. Any personal goal to beat will help make completing the schedule and doing the exercises that much more interesting. Attempting new records is always an enjoyable pursuit. If you break one, treat yourself to something special that day.

Admittedly, at 30 days, the sample cross-training schedule is quite short, especially when, for example, the marathon plan lasts four months. You may be asking yourself what to do after the 30 days are up?

Keep doing more of the same.

Plank every day. Do pushups and dips every other day.

When you can, work your biceps. If you are lying on the carpet with your children watching TV, do some crunches. Always be doing something when you have a moment. It doesn't have to be so structured. Just try to stay in a constant state of on-the-go cross-training. Stay moving and push the body. Give yourself a zero day once a week, but never give yourself two zero days in a row. Don't make up excuses for not finding the time. If you don't have time for 10 to 15 minutes of dedicated cross-training after a workout, then commit to doing just one or two exercises before you go to bed. There is always time before you go to bed. You can always find that small amount of time in your day.

The Plan: Thirty Days of Simple Cross-Training

Exercise Legend	
21s	Bicep 21s
AWP	Around the World Plank
BC	Bicycle Crunch
BENCH	Bench Press on Stab
BPU	Balanced Pushups
DC	Devil Crunch
FT	Flutterkicks
HC	Hammer Curls
HD	Hello Dollies
MPU	Max Pushups
PK	Straight Plank
PU	Pushup
SD	Seated Dips
SP	Side Plank
SR	Seated Rows
TP	Timed Plank
TRI	Triceps extensions

Week	Monday	Tuesday	Wednesday	Thursday	Friday	Saturday	Sunday
1	PK: 45 sec	21s x 3 sets	BENCH: 20 x 3	HC: 20 x 3	SD: 20 x 3	MPU: as many as possible without going to knees	Rest day
	PU: 45 sec	PK: 1 min	PK: 1 min	PK: 1 min	BPU: 45 secs	TP: As long as possible without going to knees	
	DC: 45 sec	SR: 20 repetitions x 2 sets	TRI 20 x 3	FT: 1 min	BC: 1 min	DC: 1 min	
2	21s x 3	BPU: 1 min	HC: 20 x 3	BENCH: 25 x 3	SR: 20 x 3	MPU	Rest day
	PK: 2 x 1 min	AWP: 2 min	PK: 90 sec SP: 1 min	PK: 90 sec	PK: 2 min SP: 1 min	TP	
	BC: 1 min	FT: 1 min HD: 1 min	BC: 2 x 90 sec	SD: 20 x 3	BC: 2 x 90 sec	DC: 90 sec	
3	SD: 20 x 3	21s x 4	BENCH: 25 x 4	HC: 20 x 4	TRI: 25 x 4	MPU	Rest day
	AWP: 2 min	PK: 2 min	PK: 2 min SP: 1 min	PK: 2 min	PK: 2 min SP: 1 min	TP	
	BPU: 90 sec	HC: 20 x 3	BC: 2 min	SR: 20 x 4	DC: 2 min	BC: 2 min	
4	21s x 5	SD: 20 x 5	HC: 20 x 5	BPU: 2 min	SR: 5 x 20	MPU	Rest day
	PK: 2 min 30 sec	PK: 3 min	PK: 3 min SP: 1 min	AWP: 4 min	PK: 3 min SP: 2 min	TP	
	SR 20 x 5	BENCH: 25 x 5	FK: 3 x 3 min HD: 3 x 3 min	TRI 20 x 4	BC: 2 min	FK: 4 min HD: 4 min	

five

Abstain from Astronaut Food

AT THE NEXT RACE EXPO YOU ATTEND, pay close attention to the types of food that are marketed to you. If you're hungry, expos are great places to get in a free meal, and so have at it. But instead of just grabbing at the samples and blindly stuffing them in your face, be mindful of two things: the food's sales pitch and what exactly is in the food you are eating. As Dr. Martin H. Fischer said, "A nickel's worth of goulash beats a five-dollar can of vitamins."

The Pitch

Like practically everything else in this business, running nutrition is a great place to make money. Why? Because of that age-old adage that's been tattooed on our brains: "You are what you eat." Runners seek improved performance and want to minimize their suffering on the course. They are told that if they consume a certain specialized food or potion, their bodies will respond favorably and all will be made right with the universe. There is probably some truth to this. All this nutritional research probably does produce products that help the body run faster and more efficiently when it's working hard, or recover quicker when it's tired. The science helps you in some way, but how much does it help, and, more importantly, is it worth your money?

If you stopped buying energy bars, gels, and sports drinks, if you simply dropped all those nostrums cold turkey, would your running performance decrease? Would you have a harder time completing workouts? Would you get injured? Would you fail to improve on your 5K personal record? Would you not be able to sustain high mileage?

That's the gist of this chapter: seek the answers to these questions by weaning yourself from all these expensive specialized products.

Find out what it's like to return to the basics.

The Ingredients

Not counting people with allergies and other dietary restrictions, who reads food labels? After all, they are usually located on the back of the wrapper in ridiculously small print. When you next consume an energy drink, take a gander at the label. A couple of ingredients should jump right out at you: corn syrup and food coloring (known as "artificial colors").

Corn syrup is a found in many processed foods–foods far from what you would consider healthy or "runner friendly," foods like fast food sauces, barbecue sauce, ketchup, and breakfast pastries. Some snacks marketed to runners have it, too.

Food coloring is perfected in a lab to make a drink that would otherwise look like water appeal to you when you are at your thirstiest. Food coloring does nothing for your body. It doesn't make you a faster runner; it won't help you feel better the next day. It's there to make you buy it, because you've been conditioned to associate colors with certain refreshing feelings.

Simple Food

Eat natural, organic, and unprocessed food as much as possible.

This means eating food you can find on the supermarket's periphery: fruits, nuts, vegetables, and whole-grain breads and pastas. When you feel like grabbing an energy bar after a run, instead consider an apple (carbohydrates) and a handful of nuts (protein and mono/polyunsaturated fat–the good fats). The same goes for your drinks. Conditioned to pounding a sports drink after a long run? Go for a more natural alternative, like a heaping glass of cold chocolate milk (dairy or soy–your choice).

Stay away from those health-food stores in the mall–the ones the thick-necked weightlifters frequent, the places that sell industrial-sized tubs of protein powder. As a runner, you have no business walking about in those strange stores, with their aisles of towering chemicals. Visit the farmer's market instead. Buy fresh and locally grown produce. Fill your body with fruits, nuts, and vegetables.

Weight-Loss Tips for Runners

If you have no problems managing your weight, then skip this section. However, if you're a beginner runner with some extra weight who's just starting out and would like some help shedding pounds, there are certain things you can do in addition to running a lot to jumpstart your weight loss. The more disciplined you are in following these strategies, the quicker you can lose weight and the easier your running will feel. To drive this point home, carry one of your 5-pound dumbbells with you for a quick jog down the street. Then complete the same trial run without the dumbbells.

Notice a difference?

Joint and knee pain (and eventual injury) caused by carrying around extra weight is a common excuse for heavier runners to stop running and give up on their goals. If you can quickly lose some pounds, you also lose a reason to quit.

Three Ways to Jumpstart Your Weight Loss

Follow a regimented diet program for the first 15 to 30 days of your training. There are plenty of bestselling diet books to choose from. I've had success with Dr. Mike Moreno's *The 17 Day Diet: A Doctor's Plan Designed for Rapid Results* and strongly recommend it. A program like the 17 Day Diet is intense and requires a lot of discipline. But when it's combined with running, the results are significant. The only caveat with using a quick-results diet program like the 17 Day Diet is to pay close attention to your caloric intake and your overall energy levels when you combine it with running. Many of these programs are written for morbidly obese people who aren't exercising like you are. Don't hesitate to eat more than the programs advise; you need the extra calories for your runs. Also don't hesitate to eat more complex carbohydrates (for example, pasta) than the plans suggest. Once you've dropped your initial weight (5 to 10 pounds, for example), stop following these programs and just use your running to manage your weight.

Don't eat after 8 p.m. Late-night snacking does nothing good for the body. The calories you consume then will most likely end up converting to fat. If you are starving, drink a tall glass of water to fill up your stomach. Still starving? Drink another glass. Still starving after that? Leave the kitchen and force yourself not to return there for the evening. A good way to fight temptation is to use distraction, so do something you don't usually do in the evening. Instead of returning to the sofa or your laptop, grab a book or tackle a crossword puzzle. Pick up a paintbrush and paint, or ask a loved one or friend to play a board game with you.

Stay in motion as much as possible during your day. Walk as many places as possible. If you have a dog, increase the distance of your daily walks with it. If you have young kids, take them to the park every day and play tag with them. Movement means you are burning calories. Besides walking, one way to start things out right with your new running and diet routine is to plant a vegetable garden. Growing your own vegetables gets you personally invested in your food. It's also fun eating what you sow, and the laborious process of planting and maintaining a garden is yet one more way to stay active and burn calories.

Nutrition before the Run

Pasta "Lunners"

A lot of races host pasta dinners the night before the event as a way to raise money. This is great; however, instead of a pasta dinner, races should host pasta "lunners" (a combination of lunch and dinner that would take place around 2:30 to 3:30 p.m. the day before a race). Eating a huge carb-loaded meal the night before a marathon that usually takes place early the next morning can be asking too much of your digestive tract.

Plan to eat a large meal around lunchtime the day before the marathon, but don't overdo it. Hopefully, by the time you have reached the race, you have already conducted several long training runs. Did you go to a giant pasta party the night before those training runs? Did you fill your plate 20 times? I doubt it. I'm sure you paid attention to your caloric intake the night before those long runs. You ate more than you usually do but stayed judicious about the meal. Do the same thing the day before a marathon; don't let your prerace nerves lead you astray.

Eat Like a Kenyan

If you are ever out on a run and happen to see an elite Kenyan athlete who isn't in the middle of a workout or otherwise preoccupied, sidle up to him and strike up a friendly conversation. It can't hurt can it? You'd be surprised: Kenyan runners are typically humble and will usually chat with you. Take this opportunity to get to know them. Why are they running in your country? What do they like about running here? What do they not like about running here? If you are lucky enough, you may get invited to their place for dinner.

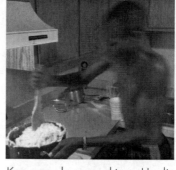

Kenyans love making Ugali. (*Author*)

If that's the case, you are in for a real treat.

Kenyan runners are fueled by *ugali*, which is maize flour (cornmeal) that is cooked with water and resembles porridge. Primarily a starch, *ugali* is packed with carbohydrates and is usually served with kale, or what the Kenyans call *sukuma wiki.*

Sukuma wiki is full of anti-oxidants and high in beta-carotene, vitamins K and C, lutein, and calcium. As far as vegetables go, it's a real powerhouse.

The ugali and sukuma wiki meal is not hard to prepare, and you don't need to go to Kenya to get the ingredients. In fact, you can find maize meal and kale at most supermarkets. If you want to eat exactly as the Kenyans do, look for maize meal that is unsifted and unbleached.

Here's how you make it:

Kenyan-style Ugali: The Perfect Runner's Meal*
Ingredients:
Three to four cups of maize meal
Four cups of water
Step 1. Bring water to boil in a pot with side handles. Do not add salt!
Step 2. Reduce the heat slightly.
Slowly, cup by cup, add in the *ugali*

*A special thank you to Toby Taner for this delicious recipe.

Step 3. Using a strong wooden spoon, stir and stroke the *ugali* to prevent lumps and ensure an even texture.

Step 4. As the *ugali* thickens, it will become harder to stir, which it is vital to have a strong spoon. Also ensure you have the ability to hold the pot in place.

Step 5. Continue to stir the mixture for approximately 20 minutes. Don't worry if some of the *ugali* mixture sticks to the bottom of the pot. This is normal and in Kenya it is often used for the next day's breakfast. Empty the ugali onto a plate and pat down to make round. It will resemble a cake, which is why it's called "African cake".

Sukumu Wiki

Ingredients:

Enough Kale to fill a large frying pan (chopped)

1 large onion (chopped)

1 large tomato (chopped)

2 tablespoons oil

3/4 cup water

Cube of bouillon (optional)

Salt to taste

Step 1. Heat the oil and then add in the onions.

Step 2. Sauté for the onions for several minutes.

Step 3. Add in the greens and tomato and continue to sauté for another one to two minutes.

Step 4. Finally add the water and optional stock cube. Cover the pan and reduce heat to simmer until the *sukuma* is tender.

Step 5. Serve with the *ugali*

At your Kenyan meal, you will notice that Kenyans get their protein from milk, which is cheaper and easier to get than meat. They also drink tea that is half water and half milk. They drop the tea leaves into a pot for brewing. Kenyans also love sugar, and joke that they put enough of it into their tea to make "the spoon stand up." There is usually no dessert at a Kenyan meal; it typically ends with tea.

Nutrition on the Run

Cheap Fuel

Sports gels, energy bars, and other science food can be handy on a run, but consider going old school with your fueling. On your especially long runs, bring something with you that will cheer you up during the hard miles. Something sugary (without chocolate that can melt), like gummy bears or candied orange slices, can provide a good boost of energy. Put a handful of them in a Ziploc bag and tuck them into your pocket. Gummy bears are especially nice for the run because you can stick them in your mouth and let them slowly dissolve. Besides candy, potatoes are great sources of energy out on the roads or trails. Boil up a pot of fingerlings on the weekend and use them throughout your running week. Lightly salt them and toss them into a small plastic bag to take with you.

Other natural fueling options include:

Dried fruit, such as raisins or pineapple

Granola bars

Crackers

Honey (buy a honeycomb and put a small piece in a plastic bag)

Jelly packets

Ditch the Water Bottle

Water bottles are burdensome. They're heavy and can throw you off balance when you're running. Hydration belts and other Batman-style gel-carrying gadgets that many runners wear are also inconvenient. They're expensive, too. It's possible to manage without these things.

Here are two ways to do it:

Position water/fueling bottles on your long-run course beforehand. Try to make these water stops mirror the ones you will encounter on race day. In other words, if you know there will be water stations at miles 3, 5, and 8 in your half marathon, place your water bottles at these same miles during your long run.

Instead of placing water bottles in advance, plan out your long runs so you can get your water for free. One option is to run at a state park and drink from water fountains or using your cupped hands at the sink in a restroom. Another option is to drink from outdoor water spigots, with permission, in residential neighborhoods. Plan your runs around your friends'/neighbors' houses and ask them if they mind your using their water when you go running. If they are runners, return the favor when they are in your neck of the woods; if they're not, do something nice for them as a token of your appreciation.

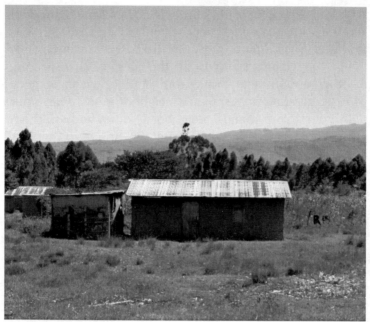
(Toby Tanser)

six

A Penny Saved Is a Personal Record Earned

THE PHOTO ON THE OPPOSITE PAGE is the boyhood home of the 2008 Olympic gold medalist in the marathon, the late Sammy Wanjiru. There doesn't appear to be any room for a treadmill. Sorry, it has no Wi-Fi. And there's definitely nowhere for you to charge your GPS watch. This hard-scrabble house is where an Olympic champion was raised; this is what he needed to run well.

Consider your own situation. You can probably get by with much less; or as Henry David Thoreau famously said, "Be wary of any enterprise that requires new clothes."

Go Run on a Shoestring

What is the real purpose of your running equipment? Running shoes serve to cushion the feet and keep you from stepping on glass shards and rusty nails. A decent hat helps keep the sun, rain, and sweat out of your eyes. Some hats, like knit caps, help prevent your body's heat from escaping. Running shirts keep you warm—so do running sweats and tights, presumably. Running shorts help prevent chafing. Socks prevent blisters and give your feet some added warmth and cushion. Shades darken the sun's light that enters your eyes. Sweatbands absorb sweat.

So if these are the true functions these items serve, why do they cost so much? And why is the running industry so fixated on creating endless permutations of these clothes every six months? The answer is obvious: job security. There is a running industry out there that thrives on selling items that appear to be continually repackaged and rebranded. It markets them to unsuspecting runners by taking advantage of their desires to run faster in every subsequent race and to be comfortable all the time. An ancillary assumption for some runners is that they need to look the part. Apparently, there are norms with runners. There's a certain running fashion out there.

The differences between a technical T-shirt and one made from cotton aren't necessarily going to make you a faster runner. This sport isn't Olympic track cycling, where every second can depend on the curve of your helmet and the quality of the lab that designed your form-fitting jersey.

This is running!

The Cost of Running: Simple Versus Complicated

Equipment	Run Simple	Run Complicated
Running shirt	Free with race entry	$30-$60
Gloves (pair)	$1	$18-$30
Socks (pair)	$1	$30-$70
Sweats/tights	$18	$30-$118
Running jacket	$30	$55-$148
Watch	$1	$25-$400
Baseball cap	$1	$18-$30
Knit hat	$1	$10-$25
Sunglasses	$1	$15-$260
Shoes	$90	$150
Approximate Total	$154	$381-$1291

"Blue-Collar" Running

Yuki Kawauchi surprised officials at the 2011 Tokyo Marathon by being the first Japanese runner to cross the finish line. In a country where professional, corporate-sponsored, full-time runners were expected to receive the accolades, Kawauchi, an amateur who worked a nine-hour-a-day job, was the furthest thing from this stereotype. "People have been telling me, 'You should do more scientific training.' . . . I don't do any of that," he says. "I think common sense and true enjoyment are what's needed. Back when people didn't have as much money they thought about their training and worked hard to get better. At some point technology became more important and they started relying more on scientific training and things like supplements and taping, and maybe they forgot what the important things are. . . . I eat whatever I like. I don't do any taping or take supplements. I don't breathe low-oxygen air. I don't wear magnetic necklaces. I guess in that way I'm old-school. I run, I work hard, and I like it. I read up, thought about what I needed to do, and found what works for me. . . . It's worthwhile spending money on things that will help your training, but spending money itself isn't going to make you better." (Larner 2011)

For most of us, this is *recreational* running. We don't need to throw our money at this problem. Leave technology to the Western elites who think it's the only way they can bridge the gap between themselves and the East Africans who grew up with none of this silliness.

At a minimum, the items we equip ourselves with, as runners, should serve a simple purpose. The simpler the equipment is, the less worry you have out on the roads, and the more money you leave in your wallet.

Leave "fashion" for other sectors of the world. Are you really out there on the roads at all hours of the day and night to look good? Do you really care what people think of your outfit? Want to be judged by passersby? Then be judged as the dedicated person going really fast down the road in the middle of a rainstorm. Be the one whom the neighbors whisper about: the monk-like runner who passes by in a tattered shirt before the roosters have started crowing. Or be the one whom other runners respect: the woman who shows up at the track in the winter wearing that same running club jacket and carrying that same shovel she uses to clear all the snow from lane one.

Embrace the "Beater" Mentality

As a child, my father always drove a "beater." A beater is a car that serves one purpose: transporting an individual or individuals from one point to another. I called my father's car a beater because it was literally beat up. My dad didn't drive it to impress anyone. It was rusty and smothered with Bondo putty. Its wheels squeaked. The heater worked haphazardly. There was no air conditioning. The passenger door took a strong shoulder to open. But the car was long-since paid for, and it got my father and his family around town just fine.

The same "beater" principles should apply to your running attire. If a bunch of layers of old free shirts keep you as warm as that expensive tech jacket, why bother shelling out your hard-earned money for it? If your running shoes don't look great anymore, if they've lost their logo and are torn in three places thanks to the day you ventured into the briar patch, but they still have a decent amount of cushion and grip on the soles, what's the rush to purchase a new pair? Try to think of your equipment differently. Think more about functionality and less about how you and it look.

Embracing simplicity with your running attire means focusing on where you get your items, how you get them, and how long you use them.

Shirts

Never buy a new running shirt. Don't go online and get suckered into microfiber this and wick-away that. Don't buy something tested in a lab with a tag that shows some sort of science diagram malarkey meant to convince you that white-coat-and-safety-goggle-wearing nerds spent half their adult lives making the perfect piece of thread for your shirt. No, don't bother. The best place to get your running shirts is at a race. Most races include shirts as part of the entry fee. And, it seems, more and more races are moving from the standard cotton race T-shirt to the all-powerful "tech" T that I'm telling you not to buy. The more races you compete in, the more running clothing you can acquire. A lot of winter races give away long-sleeved shirts, which is a great way to equip yourself in the winter. Layers of race shirts work as well as, if not better than, one lightweight, store-bought jacket, because you can shed the layers and have more flexibility with your bodily "thermostat" as you run. If you wear your shirts until they get holey, don't throw them away. What's the big deal with a small hole? What prevents you from wearing a holey shirt on a run? Afraid someone will think you are poor? Afraid it won't make you look "fast"?

This line of thinking, that you have to "look the part," flies in the face of the spirit of what it means to be a runner in the first place. There's something inherently rugged and rough about getting out there and running. You are out in the elements; you're sweating. You may be cold; you may be hot; you're always tired. So embrace these aspects of the sport. Be dirty. Be ratty. Let go of previously held concepts concerning proper exercise attire in public. There's no shame in it; there's actually nobility in not caring about what doesn't matter. Use your time to focus on what does matter—your running.

Fill a drawer at home with your old race shirts. In the morning just grab whatever lands in your hands. Don't even look at it when you put it on. If it's inside out, who cares? Maybe even cut the tags off of the shirts so you can wear them backward. Doing this prolongs the shirt's lifespan. If you are new to the sport and haven't collected race shirts yet, you can take a trip to a local Goodwill and stock up on these things. Runners who like to buy their running shirts are always donating them. And if that doesn't work, volunteer at a race or two and ask the race director if you can have some of the clothing that gets abandoned by overheating runners along the course.

Gloves

Almost every strip mall in the world has a dollar store. And despite your beliefs about the rest of the world's current trade deficit with China, you can find a lot of decent running equipment here. Gloves are probably the runner's best purchase at a dollar store. The ones you will find there are cotton and one-size-fits all. When you buy them, don't bother with colors. After some period of time, all the gloves are going to get mixed up anyway. Keep a Tupperware container near the door to your house to store them. Like your running shirts, reach in and grab two when you get ready to head out. Probably the best thing about dollar-store gloves is that they are tight. They keep your hands snug and warm.

Socks

The dollar store almost always carries white socks in two varieties: ankle length and crew, or calf, length. Buy ankle-length socks for the summer, early fall, and spring; pick up calf-length socks when it's time to wear sweats or running tights.

Headwear

If it has a bill, use it in the summer and during rainy-day racing. If it's knit, wear it when it's cold outside. Don't bother with what the hat says on it. And if it advertises something you don't care for, remove the labeling or tape it up.

Pants/Sweats/Tights

Alas, you can't find running pants at a dollar store. However, you can buy cheap new running sweats at discount chains. As with running shirts, Goodwill is another option, as is asking a race director for race-day throwaways.

Watch

A watch is a necessity during certain periods of training when you need to time your track repeats, or during race day. But it doesn't have to be equipped with the computing processing power needed to navigate a rover on the surface of Mars. A simple watch with just a timer and lap splits works great. Many dollar stores carry them.

Sunglasses

Comfort is key. Since you can usually find them at the dollar store, it's worth buying a few pairs and trying them out. Experiment with shades on your shorter runs in the event they don't work out.

Shoes

A book about running simple should surely advocate wearing the lightest shoe possible, right?

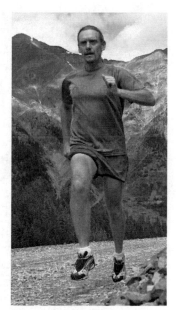

For most of your runs, all you need is a pair of shoes, shorts, shirt, and an open road. (*Meghan Hicks*)

Not this book.

These days, minimalism seems to equate solely to shoe type, or just going about with no shoes at all. There are merits to wearing true minimalistic shoes, and there are merits to wearing heavier, more-cushioned shoes. The answer to the question of which is right for you is the dreaded: "It depends."

It depends on your body type, weight, susceptibility to injury, and personal preference. I'm not against the barefoot movement, but I'm not for it either.

Plenty of other books are dedicated to running-shoe minimalism, and I'll leave you to figure out where you stand by reading them. If you want to save money by going barefoot, that's fine. However, you shouldn't do it because you've read one influential book. Experiment accordingly and apply the principles of gradualism. Also keep in mind that you aren't going to race well barefoot. Even the Kenyans wear running shoes in training, and they race in really nice flats.

With shoes, go basic and go with what works for you. Like car manufacturers, running-shoe companies have lines that range from cheap to expensive. What you get for your money is supposedly enhanced thanks to technology and features. The expensive shoes have more bells and whistles than the cheaper ones and presumably do more for your feet. I will leave what shoe works best for you up to your own preference. Don't just go out and buy the most inexpensive pair of shoes, because many factors—such as pronation (the natural rolling of the foot after it strikes the ground), motion control, and stability—need to be considered in determining what kind of shoe is best for your foot. A more expensive shoe might be worth your money. You may have to experiment.

Shoe selection is one area of running equipment where you definitely should not make a game out of saving money. You have to take care of your feet, because they are doing a lot of the work for you.

Do your homework. Learn about your pronation. Consult with experts at a local running store and have them pick out which shoe is best for you.

There is one convention worth challenging with shoes, however: their overall life cycle. Most shoe companies tell runners that after approximately 350 miles, they should begin considering replacing their shoes. They then caution you that when you exceed 500 to 600 miles, you increase the risk of injury.

This is fearmongering.

Shoe companies are businesses, and so they desire a consistent revenue stream. Accordingly, they seek to minimize the life cycle of their various models by using newly developed technology to dazzle runners who are conditioned to fear injury. Is it in their best interest to keep you in running

fortable in a Target-brand running jacket. That's fine. You know your body best, but I challenge you to try out some or all of these options and experiment with them. Make a game out of saving money with your running attire and getting by with as little as possible.

What to Do with All That Money?

Other than doing the fiscally responsible thing with the hundreds of dollars you can save by running simple—things like investing it, or paying off the consumer debt you racked up thanks to those astronomical race-entry fees—you could treat your loved one to something special. Many of our loved ones put up with this silly hobby of ours. They have to hear about our last workout. They have to deal with the mountains of sweaty clothes that pile up next to the washing machine. They have to listen to us catalog all the aches and pains we feel the day after our marathon. They get to see us crabwalk up and down the stairs. So why not put this money to good use? Surprise these supporters with a weekend getaway, or treat them to dinner at a special restaurant. They deserve to benefit from some of the rewards of your newfound wisdom.

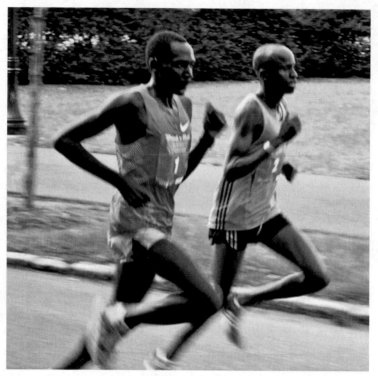

Running simple can pay off on race day. (*Author*)

seven

Race Day

FOR MOST RUNNERS, RACES SERVE AS THE FINAL EXAM—proof that everything they have worked on, all that training, all those long runs, all that sweat and doubled-over track repeats, wasn't for nothing.

Typically, this is what happens: If they fall short of their goal, they grow despondent and seek to change what they were doing. They experiment with their training week. They consult the Web. They talk to friends, experts, and just about anyone they can find in order to glean some information that will help them "right" the wrongs of their past training cycle. Finally, they venture out into the marketplace and throw money at their problem.

This chapter's purpose is to provide you with tips and strategies that will hopefully make your races less stressful and more enjoyable.

Races Aren't Final Exams!

Please don't think of races as final exams. So many of us runners do. Next time you race, just look at the faces of the serious runners at the start line. Watch the rituals. Take in the stressful atmosphere. The next time you race, think of it as an *opportunity*—a chance to run your fastest, but not a mandated exercise to prove exactly what kind of shape you are in. A race isn't the end-all-be-all, do-or-die event that most people make it out to be.

Races come and go. There's always another one around the bend. Most importantly, a race isn't necessarily the ultimate critique of your training plan and how well you executed it. If you didn't race well, it may be because your body wasn't feeling well that day. It may have been because of the 50-mph headwind in the last half of the marathon, or the fact that your mind was preoccupied with something else, like the upcoming layoffs where you work, or the loved one who's taken ill.

In order to *race well*, which can equate to a personal record or just placing higher than you normally place, you have to *be well*. Your mind and your body have to work together.

On some days neither of them shows up at the start line, and, sadly, there's usually nothing you can do about it when it happens. Like life, races are chaotic and unpredictable experiences. You just have to stay healthy, work hard, train hard, and race often. Sooner or later, you will be able to harness both your mind and your body and run well. And the better the shape you are in, the more miles and intervals and hills you run, the better your chances are that this will occur. But you also have to be prepared to plateau, and you have to be prepared to regress. It happens to everyone. Just try to stay healthy and try to keep getting out the door and putting your feet to pavement.

Here are some key strategies to consider before, during, and after a race:

Before the Race

Weather, that big messy unknown, can be the bane of a runner's existence and practically ruin a marathon. If you took part in the 2007 Chicago Marathon, when temperatures rose to a blazing 88 degrees Fahrenheit (see Davey, 2007), you can relate.

The great novelist Marcel Proust once wrote "a change in the weather is sufficient to recreate the world and ourselves." This literary gem couldn't be truer for the poor marathoner who has to deal with so many variables out of her power–things like wind strength, wind direction, dew point, and temperature.

But having so little control over events doesn't excuse you from being ignorant of what's coming your way. Don't just resign yourself to the fates, thinking there's nothing one can do about the weather.

There are these things:

Create a Wind Map

A week before a race, find out the wind prediction for the city you will be racing in. You can usually find this figure expressed in terms of direction and wind strength in miles per hour. Don't forget that the wind direction means the direction from which the wind originates. The best way to create this kind of map is to print out a copy of the course, which will likely be available online. Orienting it with north at the top, draw lines representing the predicted wind. For the headwinds miles, make the lines especially bold so you notice them when you study the map. And you should study it as much as possible. If you are traveling to your race, take it with you to examine while you are waiting at the airport or sitting on the train.

Pay particular attention to your course milestones. Study the mile markers and any relevant landmarks on the course, like a famous building or a major intersection. When reading your wind map, plan out your race and work through it in your head; imagine how it will unfold.

A good study of wind may mean asking the following questions:

Which Miles Have Headwinds? These are the tough miles, the slogging miles. You will be working especially hard here. If you can't memorize anything else on your wind map, memorize these miles. And when they come, prepare for them, mentally. Know that your pace is going to slow. You will work harder to run the same speed. During these miles, doubt is inevitably going to creep in. You may feel as if your hopes and dreams for a good race are dashed during this phase. Don't despair. Dig in—meaning get down and seek cover. Find a tall runner near you and tuck in behind him. Nearly every large race has someone willing to do the heavy lifting in the middle of a hard stretch of the course. Don't be that person. Take advantage of his kindness and draft behind him.

As you fight through headwinds, remember to make peace with the fact that they are out of your control. You may have been working for six months at a specific goal pace, developed a decent sense of comfort there, and then Old Man Winter shows up and blows your dreams away. But stay strong, for a wind-free marathon is in your future. Be patient and remain optimistic.

Which Miles Have Tailwinds? In these miles, you may have to hold yourself back. Your race can go awry in the tailwind section if you get tricked into running faster splits you have no business hitting. On your wind map, memorize these miles as ones where it's time to relax and enjoy nature's gift. Stay on goal pace here; don't try to "bank" time.

Which Miles Have a Cross Breeze? Cross breezes are painful and annoying. Usually when the wind strikes you on one side, it feels like a headwind. When studying your wind map for cross breezes, focus on which direction the wind is coming from. In this section of the race, your goal is to put a nice tall runner between the wind and yourself. Come up alongside that generous runner and run stride-for-stride with him. Let him serve as your personal windbreak.

Keep Updating Your Map

The wind forecast constantly changes. Accordingly, fill out your wind map in pencil and update it in the days leading up to the race. Study it every night before you go to bed. Ask your training partner to quiz you on it. When you are

Do as the Pros Do
The marathon team members of the Hansons-Brooks Distance Project run a 26- kilometer "marathon simulator" before their race. Brian Sell made the 2008 Olympic marathon team thanks in part to simulating the Olympic Trials course in New York City. (Larkin 2009a)

running goal-pace miles in training, visualize the wind hitting you as it will on race day. Bring it with you on the day of the race and study it all the way up to the start.

Create an Elevation Map

On race day, hills can be your best friends or worst enemies. Catch a downhill at the right moment, when you are feeling good, and you can secure that personal record or pass that opponent. Likewise if you are ready for an uphill. Although running a random route on a boring training day and discovering a hill is fun, stumbling into an 11-percent-grade, half-mile-long monster in the middle of a race isn't what you want.

You have to be ready for those race-day hills. Most large races offer elevation profiles on their Web sites. Print it out and take note of where the hills will arrive. Have the answers to these questions committed to memory:

Which is the longest hill of the race?

Where in the race does it present itself?

Based on your experiences with racing and your fitness level, how do you think you will feel when it arrives?

Are there hills before it?

How about after?

Are there any landmarks you can memorize that will help you remember the hills?

Since many courses don't deviate that much season-to-season, you don't have to wait until the week before your race in order to prepare this vital map. The moment you know where you will compete in your goal race, get to work studying the course. Then try to find a training route near where you live that best mimics the course. For example, if you are training for a marathon and you know there will be three hills approximately three miles apart from each other, set up your simulation course with the same type of hill structure in terms of distance between hills and actual hill elevation.

Another hill-related training tip is to tackle similar elevation and length hills during your End Hills workouts. Visualize the race-day hill during these workouts and think positively about it while you are gutting through it.

While reading through this section, you may be imagining only running uphill, but don't forget that downhill running can be brutal and must be accounted for in training. Just ask a grizzled Boston Marathon veteran what she thinks about that particular course and its rapid descent in the opening miles that come back to haunt the quads at the end of the race. You need to train for them, too. One way to do this is to run some of your Tempo workouts on undulating courses.

During a race, always have something in reserve for a downhill. Don't look at it as a chance to recover if you are struggling. Even though you are being assisted by the descent, your body is still undergoing additional stress as the muscles, tendons, and ligaments in your legs and feet absorb the shock brought on by the body's natural braking system.

Understand that most of your opponents on race day aren't creating things like elevation maps and practicing the hills ahead of time. So on the day of the race, many of them will be surprised when the monster hill arrives. They will probably slow on that large uphill and curse the fates as they huff and puff their way up it. You, on the other hand, have that hill dialed into memory, my friend. Your legs have been training for it, and your mind is fully prepared. It knows how long the pain will last. Take advantage of all this training and knowledge. *Make your move on the hill.* Put on a confident surge, and as you crest the hill, run through it, allocating the same effort as the course begins to flatten. Your pace will accelerate slightly, and, hopefully, your opponent will be looking at the backs of your racing flats. A few hundred meters past the hill, slow down and ease back into your goal pace.

Combine the Maps

After you've studied the wind and hills separately, it's time to put them together into a combined wind and elevation map. You can create one of these maps by printing out a fresh copy of the course map. Draw the wind arrows based on the latest weather forecast and mark the hills, using a large "D" for downhill in black ink and "U" for uphill in red ink. Where the course is rolling (sections of slight up and down), label it with an "R" in green ink, and where the course is flat use a blue "F."

With this handy reference, you can better "see" the course. Hills that are challenging by themselves may be even more challenging come race day when a 30-mph headwind blows into your face as you ascend them, so use a highlighter to note such potential trouble spots.

On your combined map, also look at the course's turns. Nearly every turn offers an opportunity to cut the tangents. Tangent cutting, running the straightest possible line in a turn, is usually allowed in a race. You can shave off a lot of time doing this. Know where your big turns are and where you might be able to take advantage of this strategy. Mark tangents with a "T."

Also on your map, examine the water stops and food stations. Try to memorize these key mile markers so you are better prepared when it comes time to rehydrate and refuel.

Write all over this combined map. Make it a worthwhile study guide.

Now Conduct a Reconnaissance

One of the most capable American commanders in World War II, General James Gavin, wrote, "If you want a decision, go to the point of danger." Gavin, who led the storied

82nd Airborne Division from North Africa into the heart of Nazi Germany, prided himself on conducting a personal reconnaissance, which meant getting a firsthand look at the situation. Though it may seem like war, a race isn't combat. But Gavin's wisdom holds true just the same.

Get out there on that course.

If you have a chance to train on it, by all means, run on the course as much as possible. If parts of the course are used in other races, volunteer for those events. Just being on the course can be a huge help. As a race volunteer, you get to see hundreds if not thousands of people tackle the same course you will be running on. Talk to some of these runners afterward. Ask them the following questions:

What did they like about the course?

What was the hardest part or parts of the race?

Which sections of the course do they recommend you prepare for when it's time for your race?

How were the hills?

How bad were the winds? Where did they feel them the most?

How was the terrain? (For example, are there potholes to watch out for?)

If you live thousands of miles away from the course, then try to arrive a few days early. Go for an easy run (or even walk) on parts of the course that you believe are the most challenging. Take the time to really experience the hill or hills. Run up and down them several times, paying attention to the current winds and where you expect them to come from on the day of the race.

If you are unable to run the course in the days leading up to the race, there's still something you can do: on the morning of the race, arrive at the course about an hour early. Starting at or near the finish line, run the course backward for 15 minutes, then turn around and run back to the finish.

Running the course backward gives you a better sense of proportion when it comes to hill length and grade. You get to examine the hill in its totality. As you are running back to the finish, you are witnessing what the final moments of the race will be like. This is the point of the course where you will be at your surliest. You'll be completely spent, throwing your arms and head wildly about. Your legs will feel like mush, and your mind will not be able to focus on anything other than the ticking clock in the distance. Perhaps at that point you will be right on the heels of an opponent, or maybe instead fending her off as she makes her final surge to overtake you. It could ruin your day and perhaps cost you a personal record or an age-group award if that small little rise on your elevation map was actually something quite severe when your tank is empty.

Best to check it out on the day of the race and know beforehand just what you are dealing with. As you jog those final 15 minutes of your test race, pay particular attention to the winds. Are they as had been forecast? Finally, look for little pockets of opportunity that you can take advantage of near the finish line. A specific example of this is a course tangent that you could cut. Any little advantage like this will pay off in these closing minutes.

During the Race

There are two words you should repeat to yourself throughout your race: "Don't panic." Remember that races aren't final exams.

If your opening mile at goal pace doesn't feel good, don't panic.

Don't panic if someone accidentally steps on the heel of your shoe and you have to stop for 10 seconds to put it back on while a horde of people pass you.

Don't panic if the winds shift on you or you accidentally drop your cup at a water stop.

Don't panic if you get a cramp.

Stay composed.

Unless you're in a 100-meter race, there is plenty of time for you to adjust to the race's unforeseen and chaotic

Do as the Pros Do
In the 2009 Twin Cities Marathon, Jason Hartmann dropped his water bottle at mile 23. Many elites would panic at the experience, but not Hartmann. He calmly turned back, picked it up, and then ran down two Kenyans to win the race in 2:12:09. "I just felt like it was important that I grab [the bottle]," he recalled. "Did it really help me? No not really, but it gave me confidence to get the fluids and energy from that. . . . In every race, you have to make a decision whether or not to go for it. I think every person has to do that. They have to decide if they are going to push forward or stay the same. At that point, I got excited and took off. From there on out, it was a race for myself." (Larkin 2009b)

dynamic. Everyone out there has to wrestle with this kind of stuff.

You aren't alone.

There Will Always Be Good Miles and Bad Miles
It's practically a given that you will feel differently during different parts of the race. Most races start with runners feeling excellent in the opening miles and end with them completely spent. However, a race doesn't necessarily have to unfold in this fashion. The bad miles aren't necessarily going to manifest themselves at the end. Your opening mile may be terrible. You may want to drop out at that point.

Don't.

Remember that bad miles come and go, and especially remember that a good mile can show up after a bad mile. Tell yourself when you're not feeling good that the next mile will be a better one.

Will it so.

When the bad miles arrive, be prepared. Know before the race that you *are* going to feel terrible and fatigued. After all, you are racing and pushing your body into a zone it's not comfortable at. With this comes the inevitable pain and suffering–the side stitches and mushy legs. When the bad mile shows up at your doorstep, greet it accordingly. Welcome it with open arms and give it what it needs, which is some sort of relief.

Slow down.

How slow?

A good rule of thumb is anywhere from 5 to 10 seconds slower than goal pace for the entire length of that bad mile. As you work through that rough patch, visualize success with it. Tell yourself your next mile will be better and that your race isn't over yet. Briefly close your eyes and work on your pain points. If your legs hurt, imagine them returning, in this slower recovery mile, to how they felt during your good miles. If your lungs are on fire, picture yourself dousing them with a huge bucket of ice water.

If the second mile is also bad, don't panic. Be cool. Slow down some more. Apply the same coping strategies. Think positively. Don't fret about how much the race cost you or how many miles you logged training in order to run this horrible race. Additional negativity will do nothing to help the situation.

If you begin to drift too far from your goal, then come to peace with the fact that today may not be your day for a personal record, but that doesn't mean you are finished as a runner or that your best days are behind you.

Run the rest of the race relaxed, and be content that you are taking part in something that is supposed to be fun. You're healthy. You're exercising. You are taking positive steps in your life. Everyone, every single runner, even the world-class elites out there, has an off day. Keep your chin up, and after the race is over, think about what you learned from this experience.

Arms, Neck, and Shoulders Relaxed

When we stress about something, we tend to tighten up—especially our neck and shoulders. Races are stressful affairs, so as you are zooming down the road or track, you may not realize that all this stress is pooling up. Your arms, too, are affected, as many intense runners clench their hands tight. All this tension can result in a cramp or a stitch—something you don't want to have to deal with, since you've got enough on your plate in a race. So when the gun sounds, remember to relax these parts of the body. Visualize your shoulders dropping and your neck staying limber. Open your hands and pay attention to them, mindful that the body's tendency is to squeeze when it's under duress.

Though I'm not much of a golfer, I once read a golf book that said the best way to hold a club is to pretend you are holding a bird. In other words, tightness and pressure do not correlate with performance. The same can be said about how to carry your hands when you are running. There's no need to squeeze.

Stop Checking Your Watch

Every time you gaze down at your watch, you are using energy and taking away from focusing on the dynamic unfolding around you. The next time you race, observe the other competitors. Most are constantly looking down at their watches or GPS devices trying to get as much information as they can. Just what are they going to do with this information? Hopefully, if you are incorporating run-by-feel "Goal Pace" techniques espoused in this book, you already know what kind of pace you are at; if you are off by a few seconds, big deal. Most races have clocks on the course. If you want to know how you are doing, use them. If you don't trust them, it's fine to wear a watch, but try to fight the temptation to consult it constantly. Use that energy to listen and look for your competitors. Also use that energy and focus to pay attention to your own internal metrics, such as rate of breathing, and how your legs and feet feel.

Fight the Urge to Quit

Races are extremely hard affairs that tax the body. When you are out there on the roads and feel like throwing in the towel, don't. Realize that most everyone out there wants to quit. The race's eventual winner probably felt like quitting, too. There is nobility in finishing a race, as opposed to dropping out. Barring a drastic injury or sudden illness, do your best to make it across the finish line.

Read Your Opponent

Racing is a lot about posturing and deception. When all things are equal, a confident, healthier-looking runner stands a better chance of winning. Remember this when you are in the middle of a race. Take a moment during your own agony to closely examine that of your opponents and try to glean some clues from them. Here are some tell-tale signs that your rivals may be in duress:

Arm Carry. How do their arms look? Are they being thrown wildly about? Did you see these runners earlier in the race? How were they carrying their arms before? Usually a fatigued runner (in other words, a runner you have a chance to beat) will exaggerate his form anomalies, which are most likely manifested in the arms. So pay attention to your rivals in the early stages of the race. When you want to make a move on them, compare how their form currently looks to how it looked when they were fresh. Wild, grossly exaggerated form is usually a good indicator that your competitor is in trouble.

Head Turning and Looking Back. My high school track coach used to say that the moment you turn around to check on your opponent, you have lost the race. That's a bit extreme, but there is some truth in that statement: someone who feels obligated to allocate the energy to turn around and see where the nearest competitor is most likely isn't feeling well. His body is hurting, and he wants to see how much he has to push in order to keep his current place. If someone does this to you in a race, see if you can manage to wave at him and flash a smile—a nice gesture that lets him know you are there and don't have any plans to leave.

Pained Breathing. A runner who's in over her head is usually pained for breath. As you close in on your opponent, listen to her breathing. Is she wheezing? Does she sound like a

19th century steam locomotive? If so, she isn't doing well and can be passed.

With this information in hand, remember that just as you are watching your opponent, you are being watched. *You* may be feeling the brutal pace. *You* may be doubting that you can beat this person, but take a moment to bluff it out. Fix your form. Adjust your arm swing. Get control of your breathing. Stop turning your head and staring at that runner who's caught up to you. There's a good chance your bluff will pay off. If you are close to the finish, your deception could discourage your opponent into thinking you've got this in the bag and that despite the Hades you are experiencing inside, you're not showing any signs of trouble.

How to Mentally Break Your Rival

There are a million ways a race can unfold. After all, races are chaotic affairs, and their dynamic depends on many factors, such as the talent depth of the field, weather, terrain, and individual strategy. But there are a few things you can do to help break stubborn opponents.

"Sit" on Them. "Sitting" on rivals means getting right behind them and letting them know you are there. Be a good sport and keep a healthy distance from them so you aren't clipping their shoes or accidentally tripping them, but still, get in there and make your presence known. Sometimes this means matching their stride. On a sunny day, when the shadows are just right, this means angling to the point on the course where they get to see your shadow for miles. They can hear your feet with each stride. Any visual cue or sound helps. Their being constantly reminded of your presence makes them worry and doubt their own ability to maintain the pace.

Make Your Move with Gusto! A surge is a hard thing to pull off when you're fatigued, but hopefully you've been training for them. When the moment is right, when you suspect that your opponent really doubts the feasibility of things, dig down deep and really explode. Your move should be *your move.* You don't want to be in a position where you will need to complete another one against the same opponent, so make your move count. Your move should make it seem like your opponent is standing still. Pump your arms and legs, and concentrate on showing him the very best of your form. Don't turn your head after you've passed him. Look straight ahead and focus on what's in front of you. If there's another opponent ahead of you, reel him in.

After the Race

After you've congratulated your rivals, it's time to start running again. Your mind and body just went through one of the hardest things they have ever experienced, and they need to ramp down properly. A good rule of thumb is to jog for at least 15 minutes after a race; 30 minutes is best. Keep your body moving. Walking is OK. As you are cooling down, think about your race. What went well? What didn't go well? Sometimes you may just be completely overwhelmed with the experience. Thinking about nothing other than how nice it is to be alive and racing is fine, too.

When you are back home, be sure to take care of your body. This means hydrating, icing, and elevating. Hydrating is obvious. Drink water first, then mix in something that will replace your electrolytes. I prefer a mixture of half orange juice and water. Carefully monitor the color of your urine to ensure you are drinking enough fluids. Icing and elevating can be completed at the same time. In keeping with the run simple approach, make sure your freezer is stocked with reusable freeze pouches that you can buy at most dollar stores. After the race, drape them over your feet and legs. Elevate your legs high enough so they are above your heart.

Now matter how the race goes, some in-depth postrace analysis is a must. When the time is right—the sooner the better after your race, when your memories are freshest—it's worthwhile to sit down and walk through the race, as well as your preparation for it.

Take your race-day bib, flip it over, and with a large black Sharpie pen, write the following details about the race at the top of the bib:

Gun time

Chip time

Overall place

Place in age group

Race-time temperature, dew point, wind speed, and wind direction

Below that information, draw a line down the middle of the bib, forming two columns. At the top of the left column write a plus (+) symbol, and above the right column write a minus (–) symbol. Now catalog what went well in the race (+ column) and what didn't (– column).

In addition, ask yourself the following questions:

What are three things I would change about the race?

What are three things I feel were out of my control during the race?

Of those three things, is there anything I can do about them next time?

Recording this introspection on the back of your bibs will pay off. If you are planning to race the same course again, find that bib and look at it. You may remember a huge hill that you forgot, or a sharp turn that isn't marked well on the course–things you can perhaps prepare for in your training. The same goes for looking at bibs from races that are the same distance as the current race you are training for. If you are going to take on the marathon after a long break, locate all your marathon bibs and try to find patterns from them that you can incorporate as you build out your training schedule.

Racing in Extreme Weather

Besides winds, two other meteorological factors you will have to account for are temperature and dew point. Of the two, dew point (how humid the air feels) can be the worst.

How to Handle Humidity

Unfortunately, there's not much you can do about humidity; it can wreck a race. This is important to note, since some people overlook humidity as a valid excuse for a bad race, opting instead to blame their performance. When the humidity is high, you simply have to make peace with your time and give yourself "toughness credit" for showing up under suboptimal conditions. One way to look at humid racing is to keep track of your personal records by dew point and temperature. What was the fastest you ran on the most sweltering of days?

Don't forget that the longer your race, the more damage humidity can do to your times. Running over 26 miles on a hot, muggy day can also be dangerous to your health. When it's time to run hot, remember: The weather pretty much affects everyone equally. Your opponents are just as hot and uncomfortable as you are. You aren't alone.

If you've been training in it, you can race in it. Unless you are hopping on a plane from Nome, Alaska, to a race in Mombasa, Kenya, your body is already adjusted to working hard in the humidity. You've put in the work in these conditions; this isn't new.

Most races are run early in the morning. So, yes, it will be uncomfortable out there, but you are probably running during the coolest part of the day.

Now that you've made peace with this experience, here are some suggestions for how to combat the brutal conditions. You can apply these tips during your hot-weather workouts as well:

Bring a cooler full of ice with you to the race and wear a baseball cap. When you arrive at the race, immediately find some shade and put a few cubes of ice into your cap. When they melt, replace them with more from your cooler. If the race isn't too long, the cooler should keep the ice somewhat frozen so you will have some ice to put in your cap after the race. If you are working out or racing at a track and there is no shade around, try to find some under the stands. Dip your cap into the ice water in your cooler. Ring it out on your singlet, concentrating on your back and shoulders.

Limit your prerace warm-up. There's no sense in torturing yourself beforehand. That oppressive heat and humidity can sap your energy. Stay in the shade and stay cool. The same applies for your postrace cool down.

During the race, look for pockets of shade on the course. Sometimes it's worth a few extra seconds to move to the side of a course in order to get out of the sun for a bit. Many races go through residential neighborhoods, so be on the lookout for kind neighbors spraying garden hoses.

After you finish the race, don't stand around in the sun socializing and backslapping with competitors. Get back in the shade and get that ice on your head.

Wear a Baseball Cap in the Rain
A lightweight baseball cap with a visor is great in the rain; it helps keeps the water out of your eyes and off your head.

Winter Racing
Racing in the cold is more manageable as a runner. You can always take actions to warm yourself–putting on another layer, donning a cap, or wearing gloves–but there's so very little that can be done when the sun is baking the world. Nevertheless, there are some winter-running precautions to consider.

Watch the Ice. The last thing you want to discover in a race is a patch of black ice while wearing racing flats. If you have encountered black ice during your training runs the week of the race, there is sure to be some lurking on the racecourse, especially since races usually take place in the cold hours of the morning. Before the race starts, ask officials if they are aware of any. You can also use part of your prerace reconnaissance searching for it. During the race itself, watch those turns and assume that ice will be present on each one. Slow down and use the straight parts of the

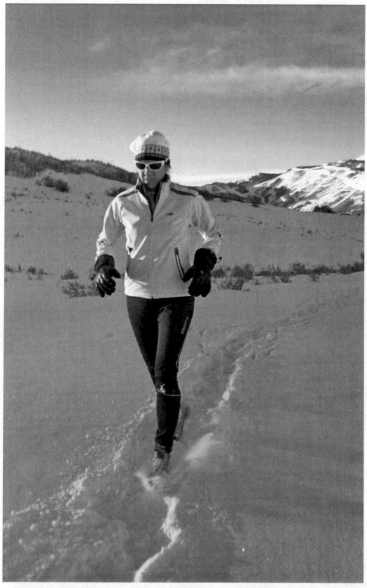

Multiple layers of thin clothing is usually a recipe for success in cold weather running. (*Meghan Hicks*)

course to catch back up to goal pace. This rule applies when it's raining out as well. Before the race, find out the last time it rained along the course, because if it's been a while, all the oil and other fluids from cars and trucks have yet to be flushed from the street, thereby making them slipperier than normal.

Don't Overdress. A good rule of thumb to follow with cold-weather racing is to be chilly at the start line. You don't want to be freezing and definitely don't want to be warm before you've started running. Since your hands and fingers get cold quickly when they whip about in the air, be sure to have on a pair of gloves. If you're unsure how to dress for the race, wear several layers of shirts. Strip down to the right layer or layers at the start, to the point where you get that chilly feeling. Resist the urge to be comfortable at the start. You shouldn't be nice and toasty. Tell yourself that within minutes of the race's beginning, you will be warm again.

Don't Forget to Hydrate. When we are cold, we often don't feel like drinking fluids. Force yourself to drink well before the race and monitor your urine color and frequency of bathroom trips. Remember that you can easily become dehydrated in the cold.

Give Yourself More Time to Warm Up before the Race. It takes longer for your body to warm up when it's cold out. Allocate an extra 10 to 15 minutes of running before the race. Start your run at an extremely slow pace. Walk the first couple of minutes. Cool down the same way.

Surge before the Start. As you mingle near the start line waiting for the race to begin, do three to five surges. Accelerate up to your goal race pace for approximately five seconds, then walk back to your starting point for one repetition. These surges get your body and mind primed to race. They also keep you warm and are a constructive way to use all the nervous energy you have flowing through you.

Take It out Slow. Even though you've warmed up properly, go out slower than usual once the starting gun sounds. Plan to run the first two miles several seconds slower than your goal pace so you can properly ease into the race.

Gird Yourself for Cold Headwinds. If ever a case could be made for drafting, it would be when you are faced with running into gusts of cold air. Find a tall runner on the course who is willing to make the sacrifice for everyone by leading. Tuck in behind that person. A better way to draft is to find a pack of runners and be the last person in the group. If you have to slow down somewhat in order to take advantage of this benefit, do so.

Finish the Race in One Piece. Just as you have to let go of your goal times in the heat and humidity, you must do the same during rough winter weather. Race for place and not for time. And even if the brutal conditions take their toll on your overall performance, remember that there will be plenty of perfect-weather opportunities waiting for you in the spring and fall.

Postrace Precautions. Bring a clean, dry set of clothes to the race. Change into them before you do your cool-down run, and put on a clean knit cap and a fresh pair of dollar-store gloves. Also, don't forget to hydrate; carry a water bottle with you on your postrace run.

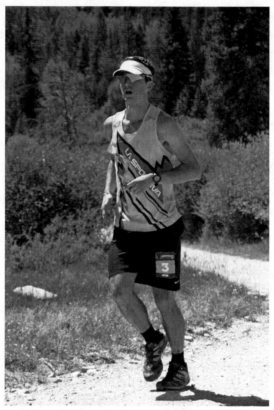

If you can convice your mind to keep going, your body will comply. (*Meghan Hicks*)

eight

Head Games

"PEOPLE MAKE A BIG MISTAKE WHEN THEY SAY, 'I need to be motivated.' You motivate yourself. I might inspire somebody, but that person has to be motivated within themselves first. Look inside yourself, believe in yourself, put in the hard work, and your dreams will unfold." I decided to open this chapter with this quote from the great American Indian runner and 10,000-meter Olympic gold medalist at the 1964 Tokyo Games, Billy Mills, because he proved that breakthrough performances are possible with the right attitude.

Though he was a fine collegiate runner, ultimately making it onto the U.S. Olympic team, Mills wasn't expected to win a medal in Tokyo. In the mix was the great Australian distance runner Ron Clarke, who had held the world record.

In that memorable race, Mills and the Tunisian Mohammed Gammoudi hung with Clarke to the bell lap. As the three runners rounded the final turn, it looked like Gammoudi would win, with Clarke a close second. Mills had fallen back, but suddenly, in the final straight, he exploded, surging far into lane three and winning the race in an Olympic record, 28:24.4, which was 45 seconds faster than Mills had ever run (see Underwood, 1964).

Most runners would have resigned themselves to taking third place that day–after all, an Olympic bronze medal is an incredible achievement–but not Mills. On that day, he believed he could beat a runner who was clearly better than he was. His body didn't win the race on its own; his mind was in control. In the race's final moments, it took charge. It made the body collect the tiny bits of energy required to win gold. The body complied because, on that day, Mills's mental attitude trumped everything else.

If you can harness your mind and body and get them to work together, you can achieve Mills-like results with your own racing. Since we all have an internal dialogue with ourselves when we are running, I structured this chapter by putting forth sample negative sentiments you may experience on your runs and pairing them with what I believe the right responses should be.

I Don't Feel Like Running Today

You aren't human if this thought doesn't enter your mind at least once a week.

Running takes a lot out of you. It can be especially rough on your feet and legs. Your body remembers this, and so you can become conditioned to resisting this prolonged bout of inevitable suffering. Throw in elements like a blizzard, heat wave, or tropical storm, and these negative feelings are compounded. The best way to combat this thought is to tell yourself that you are going to put on your trainers and run for at least 10 minutes. No matter what, you will put forth that small effort. That is the arrangement. If you start trying to make deals with yourself–crafting excuses why the 10-minute rule is baloney–then set the timer on your watch, take a deep breath, and put feet to pavement. Usually, by the time your alarm goes off, you'll be happy you're running. Ten minutes is a good duration, because by the time it expires, it will take you at least 10 minutes to return home, giving you approximately 20 minutes of running for that session—not a bad period of time of exercise when you were contemplating doing none.

One thing to try when you've lost all sense of motivation in the middle of a run is to start walking. Walking is not going to give you the same training stimulus as running, but it's decent exercise nonetheless; it's putting your legs in motion, which is better than calling a loved one and asking to be picked up at the side of the road.

Something else to think about when you have no desire to run is the nobility of any type of self-improvement. By being a runner of any ability, you are someone who is taking positive steps toward improving your health. Many people make excuses not to exercise, but on this particular day, you weren't one of them. You got out there and gave it your best. When the bad times come for you, think of this concept. And when you get outside and take your first steps on a run, listen to your feet hitting the pavement. Count the steps and think that for every step you hear, you are getting healthier and transforming yourself into a better runner.

I Just Ran the Worst Workout of My Life

Every workout isn't a test. You will show up to the track or roads on some days feeling better than you do on others. And the odds are you will bomb a fair share of your workouts. Don't panic; that's how it goes with this sport. Remember that "Race" workouts are usually done at the periphery of your abilities. You are zooming down the track at a ridiculously fast pace or you are running quicker than you ever have for a given period of time, right? The reason you are doing a workout is to take your body into a new realm—to get it accustomed to suffering; to move the pain threshold to a point that can be successfully sustained in a race. Something has to give at some point in that danger zone. If all your workouts panned out exactly as planned, you were most likely holding something back and not truly running to your potential. Occasionally bombing a workout means that you are where you need to be effort-wise. Just don't quit the thing. If you are to do 4 x 1600m, do them—even if the pace on your last rep is significantly slower than your first.

I Can't Stick with This Workout

When you feel this way, it's time to apply coping strategies. If you are giving 100 percent in a track workout, the concept of doing another one or another five repetitions can be daunting. When you reach that level of pain, the body wants to flee the scene and hide under the bleachers. So here are some tips for you when the lactic acid is pumping and you are doubled over, afraid to look at your watch and see that you have to start running really, really fast in a mere five seconds.

Focus on the number of repeats you are going to do. As you go deeper into your plan and as your fitness improves, you are going to do more repeats in each subsequent session.

If you need to do one or two more repeats than last session, then give yourself some forgiveness on your goal pace. A good rule of thumb is an additional five seconds in a mile repeat session, but go ahead and come up with your own "zone of forgiveness." The more experienced you get with track workouts, the better you will know your body and how much time to give yourself.

If you are attempting more repetitions than you've done before, try going to a track to do the workout where you can get the pace feedback you need at 200m intervals. Bear in mind, this instant feedback may run counter to the over-all "run by feel" approach that this book espouses, but there are some special cases, like this one, when checking your watch to make sure you are on target is allowable.

If you have to complete more repetitions this session, don't time the extras. In other words, if you are to do six reps and you did five last week, then your last rep, your sixth, will not be timed.

Professional Simplicity
The Norwegian record holder in the 3000m and 5000m, Marius Bakken, has spent considerable time in Kenya studying Kenyan runners, especially how their bodies adapt during workouts. "Kenyan runners have a different way of looking at things," he says. "Instead of 'no pain, no gain,' it's, 'You have to work hard, but not against your body. You have to work with it.'" (Larkin 2009c)

Wear a hat and sunglasses on a scalding track where there's no shade. Bring a cooler full of ice water and dip your hat in the cool water during your recovery period. Put the hat back on just as you are about ready to start out on your next repetition.

Bring a special treat to your workout. For a hot day's workout, it could be something like a little piece of candy (a candied orange slice, in my case), or a towel that you will wet, or a bag of ice that you will put on your head. At the end of the repeat, reward yourself accordingly. Think about your little reward as you spin around the track. Another thing you can do is make a deal with yourself—something bigger than eating a piece of candy. Tell yourself that if you stick the workout—or just complete it—you will treat yourself to a nice meal at your favorite restaurant afterward. If you're a bibliophile, you will treat yourself to a trip to the bookstore—something worthwhile that will bring a smile to your face, something worth the work.

Try to find workout partners who are doing the same number of reps you are doing. Waving goodbye to them can be demoralizing when you have one or two more reps to complete out there in the sweltering land of buzzing cicadas, while they are off to get into their air-conditioned cars and drive home to cold drinks and rotating fans.

Remember that not every repetition is going to be a strong one. Your body can be an enigma—or a stubborn mule—and you have to consider yourself lucky when you can successfully harness the mind and body to the point that you can get the body to do what it's supposed to do.

For all the other times—when, for example, the ball of your right foot hurts, or you have a stitch in your side—accept that you are human.

Run the reps relaxed; tell yourself to stay limber during each lap.

Gradually increase the pace during the repetition itself. Don't go zooming off down the track's first straight. Break the repetition into four equal parts. On a track, this means the first turn, the back straight, the final turn, and the final straight. Go out slowly and pick it up after you've cleared the first turn.

Pace the repetitions. There's no sense exceeding your goal during the first repetition and then failing the remaining five. Think about the big picture. Besides all the physiological benefits that come with interval training, there's the mental aspect. Track workouts teach you how to pace your reserves.

Say this to yourself: "One at a time." Don't do fractions and percents with how much running you have left to complete. Look at the repetitions as individual tasks. If you can get through one, you can get through them all.

Keep this in your head: "I'm trying. I'm doing everything I can to run my best. No matter how the workout is going, I'm out here doing something good for myself." Just being out on a track trying to run a workout is worthy of praise. So many of us make excuses for skipping our hard efforts. If you aren't one of them, you should be proud.

Make peace with your suffering. Running is a rare recreational sport in that it can take you into realms of pain you aren't used to being in. We in the West live such a comfortable, relatively sedentary life, and so asking your body to suffer is a bit unusual. As a human, it is your nature to avoid this kind of misery. But try to embrace it. Tell yourself that it will be over relatively soon and that your body is getting stronger because of it. Tell yourself also that you know you will encounter some form of suffering on race day and that the pain you are undergoing in your workout will make things easier for you.

I Just Failed to Run My Race Goal

Before getting into what you've already been preoccupied with since you first saw your disappointing finishing time, let's get one thing straight: Is this the last race of its type that will ever be offered in the world? Let's say you just failed to qualify for the Boston Marathon. Not good, right? But is the Boston Marathon going anywhere? Will there be a Boston Marathon next year? Put things in perspective, first.

Now, as to why you didn't run as well as you had hoped: start with the goal.

Was it realistic?

What makes you think it was realistic? Most people are extremely aggressive with their running goals. They achieve a personal record in a race and then expect the time trajectory to keep zooming downward. At some point, it's not going to keep dropping. A plateau will be reached, unfortunately. So you may be experiencing the beginning of a plateau that you may be at for years.

At this point, look back through your training logs. First, did you put in the required work? Did you take any short-cuts? Did you miss significant amounts of training? If you did everything you should have done according to your plan, it's time to examine how much goal-specific pace work your plan had and how much of it you actually completed. Count up the miles in the plan and compare them to how many goal-pace miles you actually ran in training. The numbers usually jump right out at you. How can you be expected to run 26.2 miles consistently at a 7:30-per-mile pace when all you did was put together a maximum of 5 miles at one time at that goal pace?

If you've done it all in training and your goals were realistic, how were the conditions that day? How was the dew point? How were the winds? And how about the course? Was it a fast but fair course for your goal? Lastly, how was the competition around you? Did you find yourself running a lot of the race by yourself? Sometimes you can get pulled into a personal record by others, and maybe that didn't happen during the race.

At this point, it's time to stop the introspection and make peace with the race. It just wasn't in the cards for you that day. You didn't show up with the right body because you are human and humans tend to be temperamental beings. Dwell one last time on what went well and what didn't go well. Create a list of resolutions for next time, and be done with that race. Put it behind you and move on. The history of world-class running is replete with examples of elite runners struggling one or two races before they achieve a breakthrough.

Yours is just around the bend.

I'm Not Cut Out to Be a Runner

Nonsense.

If you are capable of running, then you are cut out to be a runner. Don't think that you aren't cut out to be a runner. Don't let other people convince you of that.

Ignore them.

Don't waste your time wondering if you got the right gifts from the gene genie to run as fast as you want to run. Don't wallow in doubt about exactly where that genetic wall is for you when it comes to achieving a dream goal. Sure, genes do play a role in determining your running potential, but persistence, positive thinking, and lots of hard work may shift that proverbial wall. Just how much, I can't be sure.

Why don't you have some fun trying to find out?

Why not challenge your mind to see what it can convince the body to do? For Billy Mills, in that famous Olympic 10,000-meter race, believing in himself translated into running nearly a full minute better than his previous personal record.

If you are convinced you are cursed with a heavier endomorphic body type, then turn the negative into a positive.

Not Cut Out to Run?
One could say that American elite marathoner Nate Jenkins doesn't look like a professional runner. When he ran a 2:15 at the 2006 Austin Marathon, Jenkins, who is 6 feet tall, weighed 165 pounds. (Larkin, Interview With Nate Jenkins, 2007) That is at least 30 pounds heavier than some elite marathoners who are as tall as Jenkins. (Vigneron 2009)

Heavier runners can evolve into strong, sturdy runners. Stronger runners can usually handle more volume with less chance of injury than their brittle, nimble counterparts.

Regardless of how you look, if you can run, you're a runner, and you should be proud of that fact. Keep trying.

Don't quit.

That being said, I believe that runners, regardless of body type or goal, need some sort of fire in them to keep them running. It doesn't have to be a wildfire that's been lit by an arsonist. A fire can be pretty much anything that gets us out there onto the roads and trails. A fire can be the desire to impress a loved one, lose weight, win a bet, or simply feel we are taking positive steps toward improving our overall health.

I Don't Have Enough Time to Train

This could be the case. Running, especially marathon running, requires a serious time commitment and an enormous amount of discipline. There undoubtedly are or will be times in your life when you can't train for hours every day. Sometimes it's OK to let go of a race, especially a challenging marathon goal, because life gets in the way. But just because you give up running marathons for a year doesn't mean you have to give up running altogether.

Run when you can.

And don't beat yourself up about it. Don't look back. Don't fret. There will most likely be a time when you can dedicate yourself to tackling Boston. In the meantime, go for a shorter race that doesn't require triple-digit weekly mileage. Tilt at that longstanding 5K personal record instead.

Sometimes I Get Really Bored on My Runs

The poster boy for asceticism, Leo Tolstoy, once wrote that boredom is "the desire for desires." If this is true, when you are out on a run, you shouldn't be bored. You have desires; otherwise you wouldn't be in the middle of a cold street at 5 a.m.! But if you do find yourself getting bored with your run, ask yourself what's so boring about it:

Is your pace boring?

Is the route boring?

Are you bored because you are alone?

Are you bored because you don't think your run is doing anything for you?

Each of these questions deserves a little picking apart.

Boring Pace

You should never feel this way when you are doing a workout. If you are supposed to be working hard and feel bored, you should reexamine the pace. It's obviously way too slow. This line of thinking may get you to reexamine your goals, too. If you are out for a Rest run, then boring isn't a bad thing altogether. A Rest run is a chance to allow your body to climb back from a state of tiredness into a state of readiness. The legs are moving, the blood is flowing, and waste products generated in a previous difficult workout or extralong run are on their way out of you. A good way to cope with a boring Rest run is to head into it with other things to think about. Before you depart your house or place of work for a recovery run, create a mental list of items you want to dwell on when you are out moving at a slower pace. For me, as a writer, they can be new plot ideas to explore. As a freelance journalist, they can be new article queries to ponder. And as a father of a teenager, they can be how to deal with all the problems that come with that difficult realm. Oftentimes, on these types of runs, I get

Professional Simplicity

If changing things up, route-wise, doesn't solve your boredom problem, make peace with it. There is simplicity in repetition, and taking time in your day to return to a recognizable place may be what you need. The 2004 ING New York City Marathon champion, Hendrick Ramaala of South Africa, trains in just two places: a rolling 3.5K route in Zoo Lake Park, or at the University of the Witswatersrand's track-both in Johannesburg. (Beverly 2006)

so into my daydreaming that I lose track of the time spent on the run. Half an hour can seem like five minutes.

Try this daydreaming technique on your next boring Rest run.

Boring Route

Easy answer: change it up and change it often. Randomize it. If you are out for a Rest run, experiment with new housing developments, trails, and other environs. Perhaps bike to a place–like a state park, for example–that's too far away to run to, and begin your run from there. Talk to other runners in your area about where they run. Challenge yourself to run somewhere different once a week. If you are out of options, run the same loop you always run in reverse. Take a moment to look at your surroundings. Most of us put our heads down when we grind out miles. And if we manage to look up, our head remains fixed in front of us. But next time, actually try to pick your head up and look around. You might be in for a pleasant surprise and notice wildlife or landmarks you've never seen before.

Bored Because You Are Alone

Another easy answer: bring someone with you. Hopefully that person also wants a relaxing run. Open up a dialogue on the run. Maybe even plan ahead what you are going to discuss (taking turns?), so you aren't incessantly blabbing away into your partner's ear about your child's college application tribulations for weeks on end.

Bored Because You Don't Think Your Run Is Doing Anything for You

This kind of "What the hell am I doing with myself?" feeling is prevalent among marathoners and ultramarathoners. Anyone investing hours at a time out on the roads is bound to question the meaning behind it all. Without bothering to learn about the physiological reasons for training the body to adapt to physical stress, instead look at things with the mindset that all these miles, no matter how slow they go, are indeed doing something for the body.

Tell this to yourself over and over again during your runs when the dark moments of doubt begin to take root. In this modern day, the mind may be evolving and adapting quickly to flickering text messages, multitasking, Tweeting, and laptops with 20 browser sessions open, but the body is thousands of years behind. With distance running, the body takes a lot of monotony in order to adapt and improve.

You aren't going to get better overnight. You have to put in the time and the work. In order to make a real dent in your marathon personal record, you have to be constantly on the run, strengthening the legs and conditioning the lungs. In the end, the marathon is really about efficiency. Physiologically speaking, it's about how efficient the body is at converting your fat stores into usable energy. This efficiency has to be taught through a long and slow process that is repeated continually. Long and slow anything can be boring, but it's definitely not senseless. And that's the important part you have to drill into your head. Any successful run is progress—make that your mantra.

You Used to Listen to Music on Your Runs. Now What?

According to the American Ornithologists' Union, there are 914 species of wild birds in North America. How many of these species can you identify by call? How many can you identify by sight? Ever heard the crickets during a long run on a warm summer's night? How about the creaking sound that birch trees make when a strong wind blows through them—ever heard that? Did you know the stream along your run route makes different noises in the winter and the spring?

Get my point?

Removing those silly earphones opens up the real world around you. There is plenty of natural music out there. And if getting you to commune with nature isn't convincing, how about the safety concerns with music blaring in your ears while out running? In the past, runners have been killed or injured because they didn't hear cars, falling trees, or even trains.

We are so overstimulated these days. We crave things flashing in front of our faces and blasting in our ears constantly. We need music and get bored without it, because we have been conditioned that way.

Silence seems to have lost its virtue.

Think differently.

The next time you run without your music and there are no birds to hear—no stream, no creaking trees—just listen to your feet hitting the ground. That rhythmic pounding should be music to your ears, because it's the sound of progress. It's your source of great strength.

I Think I've Gotten as Good as I Can Get

Before you resign yourself to having reached the end of the road performance-wise, you need to really do some introspection as well as some old-fashioned sleuthing. Just like you may have done when you couldn't run a particular goal in a race, become a detective of sorts. Start out charting out all your races, and look for immediate trends to jump out:

When did you run your personal records, and on which courses?

What were the course conditions like on those days?

If you recorded your thoughts that day, consult them. If

Do as the Pros Do
Coach Terrence Mahon believes runners need to constantly
change up their training. "You are never the same athlete from
one season to the next. I think the training has to mold with
that as well," he says. (Larkin 2009d)

you didn't, try to remember what was so special about
those races. Obviously something came together for you
on those days. What was it?

You can continue to dig into your training logs looking
for clues, but don't turn it into an overcomplicated exercise. This hunt for the magic thing or things can drive you
mad after a while. At a high level, try to determine if anything really jumps out at you—such as the length of time
you trained injury-free, or the fact that in all your personal
record marathons you ran more miles in training at your
goal pace than ever before. If you can't reach any concrete
conclusions, that's OK. Most of us can't. Plateaus are probably the most unnerving aspect of running.

We all deal with them.

However, resigning yourself to the fact that no further
improvement is possible because you believe you've tried
everything is basically wishing it so. You have to change
your mental outlook. You have to stay positive and believe
that you can run faster. It's the attitude that counts here.
Keep telling yourself that your best race is still ahead of
you. On the first day of your marathon plan, as you take
the first step of your first training run, make a deal with
yourself that no matter how this training goes, you are
going to commit to doing everything you can—you will run
all the miles, complete all the workouts, race smart, and
recover wisely—with that one goal in mind.

If you can't believe in yourself, who will? A loved one
will encourage you. A training partner will spur you on and
push the pace, but it's you who are ultimately in control.
Think it so, and then go make it so. And if it doesn't

become so, that's fine, because it was one hell of an exciting ride.

Oh, No, I Have Taper Brain!

This section is geared for the marathoners out there. The hardest part of training for many runners isn't doing something like 6 x 1600m on the track, or running for an hour at goal pace; it's the taper. Why? Because if you are putting in the hard work, then you are used to continually driving yourself to the point of exhaustion. When it's time to taper, your mind and body go through a bit of shock. Taper brain sets in. Here are some symptoms of taper brain:

Loss of confidence.

Legs feeling heavy.

Loss of motivation.

Fear of the upcoming race.

Anxiety that the reduced mileage and workload brought on by the taper result in a loss of fitness.

General sense of irritability and unease.

If you find yourself suffering from taper brain, there are a few things you should do. First, understand that nearly everyone suffers from this condition. The taper is a significant shock to the system. But you need to ignore some of the body's natural impulses in your taper. After a week of reduced mileage, you may feel like you need to get out on the track and run hard.

Don't do that.

You need the rest. Drastic measures in a taper will do nothing for you other than possibly ruin your chances to reach your race-day goal. Instead, realize that what you have on your hands during your taper is a golden opportunity: free time.

You don't need to be out running, so you can round yourself out a bit as a human. If you were once a great philatelist, break out that stamp collection and magnifying glass. If your spouse has been telling you that you used to make the best homemade bread before you got the running bug, get out the rolling pin and don the apron. Always wanted to start learning Latin? Now's your chance!

In other words, do something else with your time besides fretting about your lack of running. Trust me—a well-executed taper should err on the side of laziness. You've earned the right to relax, so go do it.

During your taper runs, you can occasionally push the pace, but be careful. A general rule to follow is not to do anything faster than goal pace.

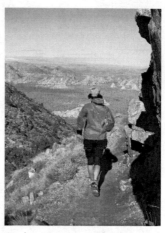

Exploring new routes is a good cure for running boredom. (*Meghan Hicks*)

The weekend before a marathon, I used to do 2 x 2 miles at marathon pace with 2 minutes of relaxed running between the repetitions. I used this final workout as a confidence booster. If my taper made those miles feel good, which it usually did, then I knew I was going to have a great race. If the miles were challenging, I told myself I especially needed that second taper week and really backed off my training then.

Simplicity in Practice

I am certainly not the first person to think about this topic. Just asking a handful of runners what it means to be a minimalist will yield hundreds of different answers. And so, to add some perspective to everything I've written about in the previous eight chapters, and to demonstrate that there isn't one answer out there to the question of what it means to run simple, I've asked four running experts to chime in on the subject: two current athletes, one former elite runner, and one coach. I selected them to be interviewed for this book because I believe they each contribute something unique on the subject.

Toby Tanser: Friend of Africa

If there's any Westerner who knows what it's like to run with Kenyans, it's Toby. In 1995, Tanser, a former elite runner born in England, had been training in Kenya. After witnessing the country's rampant poverty during that trip, Tanser was moved to take action. As he was getting ready to return home at the end of the trip, he gave away all his trainers. Tanser vowed afterward to do something more substantial to help Kenya and went on to found Shoe4Africa, a nonprofit organization that gives used running shoes to impoverished Kenyans. Tanser, who is on the New York Road Runners board of directors, now considers Kenya his second home and spends most of his time there supervising Shoe4Africa's various construction projects.

As a runner who's spent quite a bit of his life around Kenyans, what does the term "African simplicity" mean to you?

We in the West have taken the most organic and simple sport and turned it into the most overanalyzed and overcomplicated thing. In Kenya, all decisions are made purely on life matters. Kenyans tend to have a different set of rules than Westerners do. They grow up in poverty and are mentally stronger. An example of this is to compare a workout in Kenya . . . to [one in] the West. In Kenya, it's very cold in the morning. A group of runners will show up for a 20K hill workout at altitude. They jump into the back of a pickup and get driven an hour to their starting point. In the back, shivering with the rest of them, is someone like James Kwambai, a 2:04 marathoner. He's not riding up front in the warm cab. He's not given any special treatment. He's not wearing any special gear and hasn't been working out in some specialized room with a special treadmill. He's in the back of a bouncing truck freezing with everyone else. When the runners get to the start point at 1440 meters, they have one purpose: run to the top. They aren't wearing a heart-rate monitor and trying to read it constantly to understand what their body is telling them. They are simply trying to run to the top, because they need to do hill work that day. That's it.

They don't complain about it, because they have learned from an early age that complaining gets you nowhere. They have learned that life is not about complaining. It's about seeing what needs to get done and then going and doing it. After a cup of plain tea they clamber back into the

pickup truck for the hour's drive back to the camp, potholes, dirt roads, and all.

*You've run a lot in New York City, and you've coached a lot of
Westerners. What comparisons can you make between how
Westerners deal with workouts and how Kenyans deal with
workouts?*

If a Westerner has a bad workout or race, he goes home
and wants to understand exactly why he ran poorly. He
reads and reads. He gets on the Internet and tries to learn
everything there is to learn about bad workouts and how
to avoid them. A Kenyan, on the other hand, will not read
anything into a bad workout or a poorly run race. He will
just accept it. He knows that you can't win the lottery
every single day. He accepts what has happened.

It's interesting to watch Kenyans working out together.
Take, for example, a group of them completing 800s
together. Many of them aren't even wearing a watch. They
start out together, and if some can't keep up, they don't
keep up. There is no shame in dropping back, because the
pace is too hard that day. The group doesn't keep track of
how many 800s they are doing or exactly who is in the
group. They don't time how much rest they are getting.
After they have completed one repetition, they rest for a
bit and then return to the start line. If someone in the
group doesn't feel like doing another repetition, he doesn't
do it. And that's OK.

In Kenya, there is no "I'm doing this or that" with workouts. Running is part of the lifestyle. Every day isn't some
test. The Kenyans are great at listening to their body.
When they need to rest they rest. They aren't out cross-
training on their days off. They are literally lying in bed.

Do you think runners in the West measure everything too much?

Absolutely. We take everything, every little detail, too seriously. The most beautiful thing about this sport is that you
can be your best. It doesn't matter what others think. You
are an experiment of one. Other than shoes and clothes,

everything you need to run
well you have on you. And
that's where we runners in
the West start to drift away.
We overcomplicate every-
thing. We take ourselves
way too seriously. We lose
our ability to listen to our
own internal voice. Take, for
example, the cell phone.
Several years ago, I didn't
have one. I think I was one
of the last people in New
York City not to have one.
At the time I had most

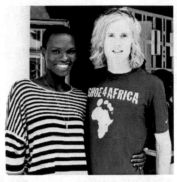

Toby Tanser has been training
and living with Kenyans for
decades. (*Toby Tanser*)

phone numbers memorized. After I got a cell phone, I forgot all the numbers I had memorized. Why? Because I had
become dependent on my phone to store them. Not my
head. That's what a Garmin [GPS watch] can do to you.
It can take away from your body's ability to measure its
own pace.

In Kenya nobody talks about miles per week. Nobody
talks about specific pace. Nobody talks about exact anything. Running is enough.

*The first example in this book is of Haile Gebrselassie. Because
he grew up in a poor family and lived in an agrarian environment, he walked or ran everywhere. This simple childhood foun-
dation helped him later in life as an elite runner. Do you have
any equivalent Kenyan stories you can share?*

Back in 1995, I was at the Iten Road Race. It was a 15K,
and all the best runners in Kenya were there. After the
start, when the runners were coming back to the finish,
there was a little boy in the lead. He was just wearing cut-
off shorts. Everyone wondered who this mystery runner
was. The boy ended up winning the race. His name was
Mark Yatich, and he went on to become a great runner,

winning the 2003 Los Angeles Marathon. He hadn't been training in a group. He hadn't been following some specific schedule. He was just a simple farm boy dressed in rags who had been running out in the woods and tending cattle all day.

That's the thing about the African attitude. They don't get these preconceived notions in their head about who is a good runner and who isn't a good runner. We look at elite runners from our country and come up with excuses why we can't be like them. But Africans look at their elite runners and say, "He is my flesh and blood. If he can run fast, I can too."

Lauren Fleshman: Track Star

There are a lot of world-class American female distance runners competing on the track, but there are very few like Lauren. Besides doing things like winning the 5000m event at the U.S. Outdoor Championships in 2006 and 2010 (USA Track & Field), she is known for her highly popular and extremely motivational Web site, AskLauren Fleshman.com, where she answers questions about running. Much of Fleshman's sage advice is in keeping with the run simple spirit of this book, which is why I chose to interview her for it.

You have been quoted as saying, "The right answer is the simple answer." What does that mean?

I am a human biologist. Nature always finds the simplest way. I work in a field that is as natural as it gets: man running. Every time I've searched for the answer to a problem or struggled to understand something running related, my aha moment has come when I've finally made it back to something insanely simple. The older and more experienced I get, the more I understand the value of simplicity in what I do.

What do "running simplicity" and "running minimalism" mean to you?

Running simplicity means not complicating things that don't need to be complicated. It is a way of looking at running and the various things that influence one's running. Running minimalism means something different to me. It means finding a way to do the least amount possible to get the biggest result. It's more of a strategy.

Have you ever run without a watch/GPS, or not cared about your time in a particular run?

Yeah, for sure. Most of my runs are like that. Any trail run or recovery day I have very little attachment to data.

Have you ever "run by feel" during a workout? In other words, have you ever practiced goal-pace runs without consulting your watch or GPS?

Yeah, Coach [Mark] Rowland has us do that throughout the year. Oftentimes we consult the watch after it's all done, but we don't look at it while the workout is in progress. This only works if you understand that the purpose of the run was to go by feel, and that all possible results on the watch are acceptable.

Do you think we in the West overcomplicate how we approach running and training? If so, why is that?

We like data. We like feedback. We like technology. We like to break things down into their smaller parts. We do it at work and in school; it comes naturally to us. I don't think it hurts most people. I do think that it is a shame not to experience running without breaking it down into data, since it's one of the few pleasures in life that doesn't *have* to be dissected. It can be a respite from all that if we let it.

You have written on your Web site that you listen to music when you run, but have you ever run "unplugged," meaning no music/electronics?

I run without music a lot more often than I run with music. I never run with music when I'm on a scenic trail, because I like to be fully present with my environment when the environment is worth being present for.

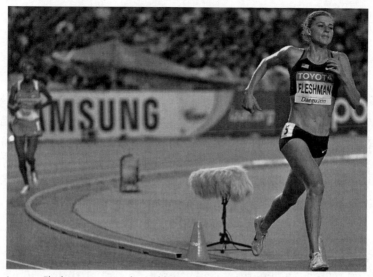

Lauren Fleshman in an elite athlete who isn't attached to running data. (*Phil Johnson, TracktownPhoto.com*)

I have spiritual and profound experiences all the time in running, which is one of the main reasons I love it. Every time I run on a forest trail, there is a point where I forget I am running and I literally feel like the boundaries between my body and the earth are an illusion. The air in my lungs comes to me as a breeze through the leaves of the trees and oxygenates my blood and fuels my cells and seems to pass through me in the wake of motion I leave behind me. Even when it is pouring rain, I am meant to be a part of it all. Running is the most obvious way that I feel like a part of the web of existence, and those experiences make me more mindful about how I treat other people and the Earth. Sometimes I am moved to tears at a vista, or a run will make me feel complete bliss. I can forget everything else and be in the moment. Listening to music on runs like this would separate me from my environment. I use music when I need help getting out the door, or when I'm doing urban running or a trail I've done a thousand times before and I simply need to get the work in.

Anton Krupicka: Ultra Champ

Watch Anton and you see running in its purest form.
Sporting a beard and usually competing shirtless, the two-
time winner of the arduous Leadville Trail 100—arguably
one of the world's toughest footraces, with nearly 16,000
feet of combined ascent and descent—is considered to be
one of the most minimal of ultramarathoners. If anyone
has something worthwhile to stay on the subject of running simple, it's him.

What does minimalism mean to you?

I guess at its core it's an elimination of unnecessary things
(material goods: which then, in the context of mountain
running, of course, often eliminates the things you might
otherwise carry with those material goods, such as food
and water). In general, it's an attempt to reduce distractions
so that the authentic things in life are revealed and more
eminently experienceable. Of course, there are several
points of debate to unpack in that statement, the most
obvious being the highly malleable definitions of "unnecessary" and "authentic."

Do you consider yourself a minimalist runner?

Well, I doubt anyone really appreciates labels. They're lim-
iting and often inaccurate, as I'm sure you're aware. I think
there are some aspects of my running that could be classi-
fied as minimalist, but there are other aspects to it that
would likely blatantly contradict such a label. To wit: my
use of a watch, my carrying of a camera on some runs, my
meticulous record-keeping, my abominable shoe collection, my occasional driving to a trailhead, [and] my jet-set-
ting ways as a corporate-sponsored runner.

You run and race a lot shirtless. Why is that?

I've always been a bit baffled by people's fascination with
this. I run and race shirtless when I feel it is hot. When I
feel it is more comfortable than wearing a shirt. Above, say,
plus-65 degrees Fahrenheit running shirtless is almost

always more comfortable to me than not. Mostly, running shirtless makes me feel more unencumbered. It's just always felt like the natural, sensible thing to do. I hated racing in singlets in college. Clammy, sweaty, chafed nipples, etc., they just feel unnecessary in the appropriate conditions. Running–especially in the mountains–is a very primal activity; I naturally gravitate toward practices that enhance that feeling.

Given the amount of technology in our lives presently, do you ever feel the urge to return to the basics with your running? What does it mean to "unplug" and run "unencumbered"?

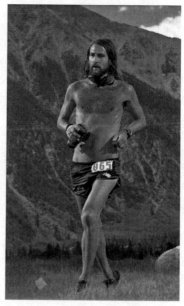

Anton Krupicka carries as little gear as possible on his long runs. (Rob O'Dea)

I absolutely "feel the urge to return to the basics" with my running. Running–and more generally, getting outside, in a wild landscape, traveling through it on my own two feet–is the primary way that I stay connected to the natural world. I was just back home in Nebraska visiting my parents for the holidays, and in such a rural environment (I grew up on a 640-acre tract of prairie hills and wooded drainages) it is much easier to maintain that connection. The way I lived there and that my parents continue to, the natural world is just so much more interwoven into daily life. Whether it be gardening, repairing a fence, felling a tree, chopping firewood, clipping a horse's hooves, etc., more of day-to-day life is lived outside, interacting with aspects of the natural world, and I find this to be hugely rewarding. Using one's body is so therapeutic mentally, and doing so in a pleasant, bucolic setting only enhances these general feelings of well-being.

So much of my day seems to be dominated now by electronic sensory stimulation–listening to music, working on a computer, watching a YouTube video, sending a text, talking on a phone–that it is imperative for my well-being that I make sure the three to four hours a day I spend in the mountains is as free from that kind of stuff as possible.

Imperative why? There's something that just feels right about it. It is definitely spiritual. It is definitely educational. The mountains have so much to teach, present so many opportunities for personal growth, and I know I would be missing a lot of that if I just numbed out the whole time I was out there, plugged into my iPod or whatever. Carrying a camera with me is such a double-edged sword because the experiences I have out there are so inspirational to me and resonate so deeply with me that I can't help but be inspired to try and share that with other people. But any time I'm carrying a camera, I often feel like I'm not able to *really see* and experience the run as readily as when I'm not worried about capturing a given shot. So I try to keep it balanced.

Do you run with a watch?

I almost always run with a watch. I can't remember the last time I didn't run with a watch–probably some race in college. I enjoy quantifying my running, to a certain extent. I don't pay too much attention to mileage anymore, but I do track volume via elapsed time. And I am always interested in my vertical gain, too. On deliberately easy or tired days, I basically never look at the watch and just hit start at the beginning and stop at the end. Running quite easily lends itself to compulsion, however, and I am as guilty of that as most anyone.

Have you ever run without a water bottle and/or fuel?

Of course–I hardly ever run *with* a water bottle and/or fuel. It depends on the weather and the time of year (summer or winter), but I have to be out for quite a long run in order to convince myself that I should carry these things. In the summer, it usually has to be three hours or more before I carry a water bottle (and then, only if I know I won't be going past any natural or artificial water sources), and four hours or more before I'll tuck a GU [energy gel] or two into my shorts pocket. In the winter, I've run five to six hours without water, only eating the occasional handful of snow. But again, above four hours, I will start carrying some GUs. For four-hour runs, I'll take two GUs, one at the two-hour mark and one at the three-hour mark. A six-hour run, I'll take four GUs, maybe a fifth just in case. Above six hours, my body starts running the risk of bonking pretty hard on only a GU/hr, so I'll take a couple extra just in case things start falling apart or something keeps me out there longer. The main reason I don't run with these things is because I hate carrying stuff when I run. It's awkward, extra weight. If I do carry water it will be one 20-ounce bottle that I will hopefully keep fairly drained and tucked in my waistband most of the time. And then, of course, less pragmatically and more philosophically, it ties into the whole minimalism thing in that the experience is definitely more enhanced the less stuff you distract yourself with. My buddy, Joe, likes to say, "There are basically two approaches: you can either go for comfort, or go for a vision."

Does running minimal give you a sense of empowerment?

Absolutely. In our modern first-world society, our basic needs are almost always very easily met. I think there is something very purposeful and illuminating and educational about putting oneself in a situation where [things] get a little desperate and you have nothing but your own strength and will to get you through it. It is a very privileged and bourgeois position to be in–to be willfully denying oneself creature comforts–but I don't think that negates the fact that we can learn a lot from being in such situations; that these situations are unique opportunities for personal growth. There is a very Emersonian radical self-reliance aspect to my running in the mountains that has definitely become a foundational cornerstone to my identity and psyche.

Do you believe that running in general has become overcompli-cated and that Western runners are overloaded with too much information and feedback?

I don't really know. I don't think it really has to do too much with "information and feedback." Though I think there is something to be said for learning to be more intuitive about listening to your body rather than always relying on an instrument (heart-rate monitor, GPS, etc.). I think the more concerning issue is that there are probably sectors of Western runners who, instead of putting in the hard work of actually just getting out and *running*, try to identify themselves with the running tribe by instead buying all the key material signifiers that have been marketed to them as being required to be part of the clan: FiveFingers, Hokas, fuel belts, compression everything, visors, sunglasses, GPS this, heart-rate-monitor that, etc., etc. Plugging into consumer culture is way easier than doing the hard work of actually learning something about yourself, what your tastes are, what *your* ideas are, what makes *you* feel whole. It's much easier to buy into the pre-set program. There are whole sectors of running society that I don't identify with at all. Instead, I identify with and am inspired by anyone who is outside interacting with their landscape in an authentic, intentional, and inspired fashion, whether they be climbers, skiers, alpinists, surfers, slack-liners, cyclists, farmers, kayakers, hang-gliders, BASE jumpers, etc. I am inspired when the activity becomes more about immersion and art than about numbers and performance. It just so happens that the people who are most tuned in to the former in the mountains often put up the most impressive numbers and performances, too.

Do you have any success stories you can share regarding your own experience with minimalism?

Every single day that I'm able to get out up in the mountains and be affected in a positive way by the experience–that's absolutely a success. This morning was a huge success. I woke up to a raging wind that, had I just stayed inside, I would hardly have realized was even occurring. As I jogged up toward the trailhead, a flaming, spectacular sunrise reflected off the Flatirons–one of those moments of beauty that evokes an internal feeling that can't really be related–and then for the next 35 minutes I post-holed through knee-deep snow, scrambled on all fours over and past giant slabs of rock, nearly lost my vision to exertion and hypoxia until I was finally on the summit, 3,000 feet above the town below, where I enjoyed a few minutes of silent contemplation before bombing back down the mountain on a mix of icy trail and techie cross-country terrain, where I achieved a few occasional fleeting stretches of what felt like absolute union between my footwork, my rate of descent, and the surrounding terrain. One hour and forty minutes later, and I'd had an enriching and satisfying enough experience–even though I was tired most of the time–that it will take a whole lot today for anything to truly piss me off.

Do you think Western runners could be better runners if they ran with fewer encumbrances and instant feedback?

I guess it all depends on what "better" means. It depends on what a given runner's goals are. What do they want to get out of the activity? *Why* are they running? Obviously, I think it is easier to be conscious, present in the moment, more open to inspiring moments of beauty when you have fewer encumbrances. But those are the reasons I run, not necessarily why everyone else runs or even should run.

Most of all, I think it is important that people simply get out there, move around, refamiliarize themselves with the fact that they actually *have a body*. And if it takes a few techno gizmos to motivate that, then fine. It's just not what I prefer with my running.

Brad Hudson: Coach

Brad is one of the best American distance coaches out there. As an athlete, he was a 2:13 marathoner and a multiple All-American in college. As a coach, he's a constant resource for numerous Olympic-caliber runners, ranging from middle-distance to the marathon. Brad is the coauthor of a great book, *Run Faster from the 5k to the Marathon: How to Be Your Own Best Coach.*

When you hear the word "minimalism," what thoughts come to mind?

To me, it means being a little more stripped down. Feet do naturally what they do, and, like everything, I look at everyone individually. I do have a lot of people that I coach who run in racing flats and other minimalism type of shoes. As with anything, I think you gradually have to build it in—not to start running barefoot but to see what works for you. It's the same as with your training; you need to find the best solution for you. The bottom line is to keep people healthy. With that said, I've had a lot of success with people. I had one athlete who tried everything from orthotics to seeing every doctor. He was always injured. He went to a minimalist shoe and is running 120 miles a week and has never really been injured or missed a day. But like anything, minimalism must be taken with a grain of salt and looked at methodically. I worked at a running store, and people would come in and go right to minimalism. I saw a lot of problems because they weren't gradually building it in. Like anything, you need time to strengthen your feet and get used to it, but I am, by no means, 100 percent minimalist, because I've seen people have negative results with it. From a philosophy standpoint, it makes complete sense as long as people take the time to do it properly and at their own level.

You answered the last question in terms of minimalism regarding footwear, but what are your thoughts about simplicity in running?

Even though I'm very analytical when I look at everything, I try to make things as simple as possible for the athletes because they like it better. And it's just a smarter way of doing things as opposed to being gauged in with paces, VDOT [a term coined by coach Jack Daniels to predict equivalent performance at different racing distances], etc. Really, the main thing they have to learn is to feel. The difference between the Kenyans and U.S. athletes is that they, the Kenyans, go a lot on how they feel on their paces. It doesn't mean they don't push themselves, but it means they listen to their bodies and internal clocks a little more— their own biofeedback, their own breathing, and their own respiration.

As a coach, I like this GPS stuff because I don't have to wheel everything out, but I don't like my athletes wearing a GPS watch every day. They start to analyze how they felt at certain paces when it means nothing. They push too much sometimes during the beginning of a run because they are pacing their whole run rather than just warming up. You'd be surprised how slow some of these elite runners run during the first 10 to 15 minutes of their workouts. That is a good thing. It prevents injuries. I'd much rather have them doing that then saying, "Well, I'm only running 9:00 pace right now." I definitely believe in keeping things pretty simple. The number one coach is yourself and how you are feeling. It doesn't mean that every person is going to push themselves. There are times when I think you have to override your own internal clock, but for the most part, people can do so much better by just listening to their body and not being tied to what there are supposed to do.

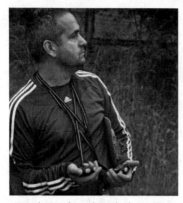

Coach Brad Hudson believes running technology is not something to obsess about. (Kevin Danaher)

Do you think that the Western running world is overdependent on technology?

Oh yeah, for sure. It's good for business, for our sport, because there are other things that can be tied into running. I think there's a time and a place for the technology, but I do think that we are too tied to it on our easy days and on our days that are meaningless.

As a coach you talked about keeping things as simple as possible with your athletes. Can you provide some examples?

At the end of the day, I have athletes that have been injured, and I help them by just looking at what they need to do and not make things too overcomplex. I have an athlete in Seattle that was having a lot of plantar fasciitis problems. The speed work was tending to aggravate him, and he's going into the Olympic marathon trials in the best shape. All I did was say, "Let's look at the marathon. What do you need to be specific?" I kept pace-specific runs in his training, and he's in the best shape of his life. I always make things simple–even when I look at things technical. I look at making things as easy as possible for the athlete.

Do you ever tell your athletes to not wear a watch or not look at a watch in training?

Yeah, for sure. At the end of the day, I assign paces. As we get more into the specific period, I'm more into timing. I'm a little more into seeing where they are. I'm adamant that they run paces, and I get a little bit of an idea where they are. For the most part, in the fundamental period, I strongly believe that people should just run how they feel. Forget their watch. They need to learn what 10K is and what threshold is. If you really listen to yourself you can figure it out. I've had so many people that just listen to their body–even wearing a heart-rate monitor–and then they get tested. They can easily guess within one or two beats what their threshold is. That tells you a lot–it tells you that if you just listen to yourself, you can learn as much as this testing, even more.

Let's say I'm a new runner and I went and bought my new GPS watch and my other devices, but I want to wean myself off of it. Would it be good to do it on a recovery day first, as opposed to a workout day?

Yeah, I have a group of elite athletes that I have training for the [U.S. Olympic] Trials. I'm fine with them working out together one day a week and pushing themselves. You will lessen your mistakes, and your margin of error will be so much smaller, if you run hard on your hard days and run by yourself on your easy days. The biggest mistake I've seen with elites is when they all train together every single day, because they are competitive, and someone is always feeling good. One thing for sure is you could give everyone 10 x 1K, the same workout, but how they recover is so much different. I have some people that can spring up the next day and run consistently. A lot of people may need two or three days of their own recovery. The biggest thing I can say is to wean themselves off the technology on the days that are the most meaningless, which are the days when they have to go off feel. I think a lot of injuries are caused by not being warmed up. Some of that can be them being obsessed with their average pace the whole run. Every run should be some sort of progression run, because you need to warm up. The more volume you run and the harder you train makes it an even bigger factor.

You mentioned African runners being simpler. Do you think that is a contributing factor to them being better runners than the rest of the world?

Yes. . . . [T]hey are much more active than we are in the U.S. I'm not against technology by any means, but I think it's something that needs to be in its right place and not obsessed about. I've seen so many athletes get upset in their workouts because they aren't hitting the paces. And that's caused by their GPS telling them something, or because it's a windy day, or there are horrible conditions. The bottom line is that they have to listen to their body. It's the same way in a race. You are never going to get perfect conditions. It's OK at times to worry about pace and the technology of how they are doing and the measurement of their exact performance, but those instances should be few and far between.

ten

Your Questions, My Answers

AT THE BEGINNING OF THIS BOOK, I tried driving home the point that this isn't necessarily a rigid guide. After all, rigidity does not equal simplicity.

So please get creative. Apply your own mantras, beliefs, and personal situations to how you approach running and how you schedule your training. This isn't an equation to solve or a book to balance; it's a mystery to comprehend.

Enjoy the experience. And remember that you don't need to be a world-class athlete or an elite coach to know how to run. You know more about the sport than you realize.

I wrote this book to get you to think differently about your running. It doesn't matter if you are a first-time marathoner or someone who's run Boston for 20 consecutive years. When you put the book down, be vigilant of the running industry out there. Don't get sucked into believing that science and gadgets are all you need to close the performance gap between what you want to achieve and what you have achieved.

Hard work and the right attitude will suffice.

In parting, I tried to come up with some questions you may have and my answers to them. I tried putting myself in your shoes and asking myself things I may not have done the best job of addressing earlier. I'm sure there are some inconsistencies and inaccuracies that I inadvertently overlooked, and for them I apologize.

How fast should I run on my Rest days?

That's a trick question, because you shouldn't be measuring pace on your Rest days. A good rule of thumb is to run so slow you can carry on a relaxed conversation with someone the entire way. If you are struggling in any way during a Rest day, you are overdoing it and should slow down until you get that enjoyably comfortable feeling. You can walk if you want.

How can I work other races into the schedule?

Tune-up races are excellent ideas, since they afford you the ability to compete and better learn about yourself as a racer. Essentially, anytime you have a Race day on your training schedule, feel free to substitute a real race in its place. But try not to race too frequently. Just how often is too often depends on the length of the tune-up races and how you respond physically to them. Another thing to consider is that frequent racing at distances shorter than your goal race can get in the way of your Goal-Pace workouts. Take the middle path with races; do them as you see fit, but don't get carried away. And definitely don't do them when you are supposed to be doing Just Run or Rest runs.

I've found that it's hard for me to quit using my electronics cold turkey. Can I slowly wean myself off my gadgets?

This isn't something serious like a substance-abuse problem. Electronic gadgetry and listening to music while running are things you should be able to get rid of fairly quickly. However, if you need more structure on how to do this, try the following three-week approach:

For the first week of your electronics-weaning period, permanently give up all biofeedback devices (for example, heart-rate monitors), and don't wear a GPS watch during any of your Race workouts.

In the second week, permanently give up your GPS watch, and don't listen to your music during your Race or Just Run workouts.

In the third week, permanently give up your music and begin to truly run simple.

If you find yourself still using your gadgetry after three weeks, it's time to take the tough love approach and lock them up, as discussed in chapter 2.

I got injured. How do I start up the schedules again?

It depends on your injury. If you are sidelined for less than a week, you shouldn't do anything to the schedule. Just keep plugging away on the schedule. If you are out for more than two weeks, you should alter your schedule. Use the principles outlined in chapter 3 to reset things.

I'm an older runner (over 40) who is just starting out. Should I do anything different?

Not really. The only thing to take into account as an older runner is that it may take longer for you to recover after a harder workout or a long run. As you build out your schedule, put in an extra day, or maybe two, of Rest runs during the week..

Why doesn't this book differentiate between the sexes in the training schedules?

The schedules are designed to give you a rough example of how to incorporate and integrate all the training principles in the book. They aren't to be followed like a cooking recipe. I don't believe these schedules are universally applicable, and they might not make sense to you. If that's the case, then study the concepts behind the schedules and develop your own.

Why aren't there any Goal-Pace runs in the 5K/10K schedules?

These races, 5Ks in particular, are fast. Your Goal-Pace work is covered when you are doing your tempo runs and track repeats in the schedule.

Can I run longer for warm-up/cool down on my Race days?

I rarely discourage people I coach from running. Go for it. Just don't overdo things. The purpose of your Race days isn't to build up a ton of time on your feet, but to be ready to step up on the track or trails to run your workout. In other words, don't compromise your workout by over-achieving with your warm-up. Be cautious during your cool down. Even if you are feeling good, remember what you just put your body through.

Can I splurge on racing flats?

Absolutely. Running simple doesn't mean racing stupid. Shoe companies manufacture some fantastic flats that can cut down on your times due to their lightweight nature and design. Go for it.

Dollar-store socks cause blisters. What can I do about that?

Don't buy something that makes you uncomfortable and causes blisters just for the sake of simplicity. But do think about low-cost alternatives before being duped by "sports science." If a dollar store doesn't have what you need, maybe a discount store will. Experiment with frugality before you throw money at the problem.

For safety reasons, I carry my phone with me when I run. Is that OK?

Absolutely. Safety and security always come first. Having a phone with you for emergency purposes can be a good thing, especially on a long run, or a run in a strange or uncertain locale. However, I recommend that you store it out of sight and not check your messages, Facebook news-feed, or listen to music on it while you are running. Have it on you, but don't meddle with it at all. Except for matters of safety and security, stay off the grid.

I have a friend who owns a local running store. You tell me to buy my running gear at the dollar store. This means not giving her my business. Can I shop local?

Absolutely. Please support your local running businesses–even if it means buying marked-up items from them. They need your business and deserve your money. They also do wonderful free things for your running community, like organizing races and hosting seminars. But strike a balance. Perhaps buy your shoes from them, but get your winter hat and gloves at the dollar store. As for the running industry, it's doing just fine; I sincerely doubt this book will hurt it.

I like to run on a treadmill, and the only way to do that is by joining a gym–something you tell me not to do. What should I do?

Why do you need to run on a treadmill? If it's snowing outside with 40-mph gusts of arctic air and you hate running in that kind of madness, then sorry–get used to running in it. Deal with the elements; they are part of the equation and can't be ignored in training. You don't get an alternative on race day, do you? That being said, there are some valid reasons to join a gym and jump on a treadmill; here are a few: I was a single dad for a few years. My daughter was too old and too big for me to push her around in a jog stroller. She was also too young for me to leave her alone at home when I was running. To resolve this dilemma, I saved up and bought a treadmill that I kept in my basement. I ran on it at night after I had put my daughter to bed. I can see the case for someone in a similar position needing to join a gym for the childcare benefits, or doing as I did and buying a treadmill for the home. Treadmills are also OK to use when you are traveling and not able to run in a strange location. And they are also OK for people who don't have access to hills.

I don't have a golf course or a track or a hill where I live. What should I do?

If you can't complete tee-to-green workouts, try the alternatives I provide in chapter 3. If you don't have a track near you, do your track workouts on the road using measured landmarks. And in the event you live in Kansas, there are several ways to try to simulate the resistance of a hill: find a treadmill and use the elevation setting on it, or run on sand, or push a jogging stroller. You can also do hill-type workouts at a large stadium on stairs or even up and down stadium ramps.

None of the training schedules mention running twice a day. Can I double?

This book was written based on not breaking up the training in any manner. Doubles can have their place for serious marathoners, but I'll leave that subject to other books and better-qualified experts. Just know that what you need to do in training to run well can be accomplished by running once a day. After all, doubling increases the complexity of your day. You have to make the time to not only run twice, but possibly shower twice and get changed into and out of running clothes twice. Doubling is not running simple.

Nothing in this book tells me when it's OK to take a zero day. Can I take a day off every now and then?

You know your body better than I do. If you are feeling like you need a zero day, then take it. But before doing so, I think you should try to persuade yourself to do some sort of running. Instead of not running at all, consider one of the Rest alternatives like walking. As for people conditioned to taking a zero day once a week: if you follow the principles outlined in this book, I don't think you'll need that much rest. When done properly, your Rest runs should get you prepared for the higher mileage of your Just Run days and the pace stress of your Race days.

In the book you've interviewed a professional ultramarathoner, but you don't offer any sample ultramarathon training schedules. You don't even address ultramarathon training. Why is that? I'm preparing for my first ultramarathon. What do I do?

There's no reason you can't apply the run simple principles outlined in chapter 3 to develop your own ultramarathon training plan. I didn't include a sample ultra schedule because finding the time to properly prepare for something like a 100-mile race entails a lot of customization (and juggling) of your personal schedule. If you are going to put together your own ultra plan, I suggest completing more Just Run days at the expense of Race days. I believe that speedwork is a necessary component in any running schedule, but there's no need to be doing twice weekly track repeats or shorter, quicker tempo runs as a nascent ultra runner. Instead, get as much time on your feet as possible. Every week, gradually increase the length of your long run, and try to work in one or two additional especially long runs every week.

The sample training schedules lump together 5K and 10Ks. The 10K is twice the distance of the 5K. Why are these races treated equally?

To keep the book from becoming another "Run Complicated" variant, I opted not to differentiate between the 5K and 10K in the sample schedules. With the volume of 400m and 800m track repeats in the 5K/10K schedules, I've admittedly favored the 5K. But the schedules still have 10K-type tempo runs and a fair amount of long runs. If you are training for a 10K and don't like what you read, incorporate a few longer track repeat days, like 1200m or 1600m reps, into your plan.

This book is called Run Simple, *yet in the racing chapter it suggests creating complex-looking wind and elevation maps and doing detailed analysis of the course. How is that kind of activity in keeping with the principles of not complicating things outlined in other parts of this book?*

Just as running simple doesn't mean racing stupid, it also can mean not racing ignorant. If you are spending large chunks of your life training for a certain goal race, then there is nothing wrong with preparing for it properly. Other than reading the weather forecast and cross-referencing it against a course-elevation profile, there isn't much required of you before the race. I'm not telling you to wear an anemometer, or take elevation measurements during your runs; I'm telling you that you don't want to be surprised by the elements on race day.

Do you have anything else to say before I close the book?

Let me leave you with a few gems that I hope you can carry with you for a long time:

No matter what you take away from reading this, please remember to always commit to looking at your running differently.

Disregard external biofeedback and all the cyber chatter out there. Don't let anyone dial you into a group or category. No stereotypes allowed. Just because your first marathon was four hours doesn't mean you can't run an Olympic-Trials-qualifying time in four years. Who said you couldn't? The peanut gallery on a bulletin board? Who are they to you? Nobody.

Running may seem like a complex activity; it's not. The more you do it, the better you can become. Keep at it. There is no substitute for hard work. Put in the mileage and put in the workouts. Keep telling yourself you can achieve your goal. If you fall short, if you stumble, which you will, because you are human, stay optimistic. And stay grounded: it's the possibility of running your personal record that should excite you the most—not actually pulling it off.

Learn to put your mind in the driver's seat. So much is written about the body for runners—how to physically run longer and faster—but so little is written about the mind. Remember what Billy Mills was able to achieve when he believed in himself.

Always RUN SIMPLE.

Bibliography

American Ornithologists' Union. 2011. *Checklist of North American Birds*, August 8. Retrieved January 25, 2011, at http://www.aou.org/checklist/north/index.php.

Beverly, J. 2006. "Street Fighter: Hendrick Ramaala Acts Like Just One of the Guys—but Don't Let That Fool You." *Running Times*, November.

Davey, M. 2007. "Death, Havoc and Heat Mar Chicago Race." *New York Times*, October, 8. Retrieved February 14, 2012, at http://www.nytimes.com/2007/10/08/us/08chicago.html?pagewanted=all.

Ferstle, J. 2012. "Peter Snell: Gentleman, Athlete, Scholar." *Running Times*, February/March. Retrieved February 2, 2012 at http://www.runningtimes.com/print.asp?articleID=25055

Larkin, D. 2007. *Interview With Nate Jenkins*. New York Road Runners, October14. Retrieved February 11, 2012, at http://www2.nyrr.org/races/pro/interview/2007/natejenkins101907.asp.

———. 2009a. *Brian Sell Interview*. Roads, Mills, Laps, October 2. Retrieved February 28, 2012, at http://www.roadsmillslaps.com/RML/blog/Entries/2009/10/2_Brian_Sell.html.

———. 2009b. *Jason Hartmann Interview*. Roads, Mills, Laps, October 23. Retrieved February 10, 2012, at http://www.roadsmillslaps.com/RML/blog/Entries/2009/10/23_Jason_Hartmann.html

———. 2009c. *Marius Bakken Interview*. Roads, Mills, Laps, September 29. Retrieved February 8, 2012, at http://www.roadsmillslaps.com/RML/blog/Entries/2009/9/29_Marius_Bakken.html.

———. 2009d. *Terrence Mahon Interview*. Roads, Mills, Laps, October 9. Retrieved January 20, 2012, at http://www.roadsmillslaps.com/RML/blog/Entries/2009/10/9_Terrence_Mahon.html.

———. 2010a. *Proceed With Caution: Exclusive Interview With Ray Treacy.* Competitor, August 30. Retrieved February 28, 2012, at http://running.competitor.com/2010/08/features/proceed-with-caution-exclusive-interview-with-ray-treacy_12668.

———. 2010b. *Tim Broe: Godfather of the Grinders.* Roads, Mills, Laps, August 22. Retrieved March 1, 2012, http://www.roadsmillslaps.com/RML/blog/Entries/2010/8/22_Tim_Broe__GodFather_of_The_Grinders.html.

Larner, B. 2011. "Working His Way to the Top: How Motivated Civil Servant Yuki Kawauchi Beat the Japanese System (and Ran 2:08)." *Running Times,* October.

Noakes, T. 1991. *Lore of Running.* Champaign, IL: Human Kinetics.

Underwood, J. 1964. "We Win the Five and Ten." *Sports Illustrated,* October 26. Retrieved February 2, 2012, at http://sportsillustrated.cnn.com/vault/article/magazine/MAG1076522/index.htm.

USA Track & Field. n.d. *Athlete Bios.* Retrieved February 2, 2012, at http://www.usatf.org/Athlete-Bios/Lauren-Fleshman.aspx.

Vigneron, P. 2009. "Grinder: Nate Jenkins Is a Hero for All Runners With More Grit Than Genetic Gifts. *Running Times,* July/August.

White, J. 2011. "Born to Run: Haile Gebrselassie Interview." *The Telegraph,* March 17. Retrieved February 2, 2012, at http://www.telegraph.co.uk/sport/othersport/athletics/8373361/Born-to-run-Haile-Gebrselassie-interview.html.

Index